Lung Cancer

Despite the worldwide drive to increase awareness of the risks of smoking, lung cancer remains a global problem.

A multidisciplinary team approach is now considered the most effective way to manage lung cancer. Imaging plays a central role in this multidisciplinary approach; this is reflected in the present volume.

Individual chapters focus on imaging (including screening, diagnosis of symptomatic cases and staging) pathology and treatment options in lung cancer. Due to recent interest in the potential role of PET for a variety of malignancies, a separate chapter is devoted to this technique.

Each volume in *Contemporary Issues in Cancer Imaging* is coordinated by an expert guest editor with contributions from all members of the multidisciplinary team, bringing together expertise from many specialties to promote the understanding and application of modern imaging in patient management.

Sujal R. Desai is a Consultant Radiologist at King's College Hospital, London.

Contemporary Issues in Cancer Imaging

A Multidisciplinary Approach

Series Editors

Rodney Reznek
Cancer Imaging, St Bartholomew's Hospital, London

Janet Husband
Diagnostic Radiology, Royal Marsden Hospital, Surrey

Lung Cancer

Sujal R. Desai

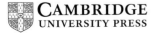

CAMBRIDGE
UNIVERSITY PRESS

CAMBRIDGE UNIVERSITY PRESS
Cambridge, New York, Melbourne, Madrid, Cape Town, Singapore, São Paulo

Cambridge University Press
The Edinburgh Building, Cambridge CB2 2RU, UK

Published in the United States of America by Cambridge University Press, New York

www.cambridge.org
Information on this title: www.cambridge.org/9780521872027

First published 2007

Printed in the United Kingdom at the University Press, Cambridge

A catalogue record for this publication is available from the British Library

Library of Congress Cataloging-in-Publication data

Lung cancer / [edited by] Sujal Desai.
    p. ; cm. -- (Contemporary issues in cancer imaging)
  Includes bibliographical references and index.
  ISBN-13: 978-0-521-87202-7 (hardback)
  1. Lungs–Cancer. I. Desai, Sujal, 1962-II. Series.
  [DNLM: 1. Lung Neoplasms. WF 658 L96065 2006] I. Title. II. Series.

  RC280.L8L76535 2006
  616.99'424--dc22
                                                              2006031970

ISBN-13 978-0-521-87202-7 hardback
ISBN-10 0-521-87202-2 hardback

Contents

Colour plate section appears between pages 20 and 21

Contributors

Shahreen Ahmad, B.SC., M.B.B.S., M.R.C.P., F.R.C.R.
Guy's, King's and St Thomas' Joint Cancer Centre
Department of Clinical Oncology
St Thomas' Hospital
London, UK

Zelena A. Aziz,
Department of Radiology
St Bartholomew's and the Royal
London Hospital
London, UK

Andrew Chukwuemeka, M.D., F.R.C.S.
SELCN Lead for Lung Cancer Research
Guy's, King's and St Thomas' Cancer Centre
London, UK

Gary. J. R. Cook, F.R.C.R., F.R.C.P.
Department of Nuclear Medicine and PET
Royal Marsden Hospital
Sutton
Surrey, UK

Sarah. J. Copley, M.D., M.R.C.P., F.R.C.R.
Department of Radiology
Hammersmith Hospital
London, UK

Thomas E. Hartman, M.D.
Department of Radiology
Mayo Clinic
Rochester, MN, USA

Sayed A. M. Z. Jafri, M.B.B.S., M.R.C.S.
Department of Radiology
Hammersmith Hospital
London, UK

Thomas. B. Lynch, F.R.C.P.
Department of Nuclear Medicine and PET
Royal Marsden Hospital
Sutton
Surrey, UK

Michael T. Marrinan, F.R.C.S.ED.
SELCN Lead for Lung Cancer Research
Guy's, King's and St Thomas' Cancer Centre
London, UK

Sabine Pomplun, M.SC., M.D., M.R.C. PATH
Department of Histopathology
King's College Hospital
London, UK

Joseph Prendiville, PH.D., MB., B.C., B.A.O., F.R.C.P.
SELCN Lead for Lung Cancer Research
Guy's, King's and St Thomas' Cancer Centre
London, UK

Alistair Ring, M.A., B.M., B.CL.,
M.R.C.P., M.D.
SELCN Lead for Lung Cancer Research
Guy's, King's and St Thomas'
Cancer Centre
London, UK

Pallav Shah, M.D., F.R.C.P.
Royal Brompton Hospital
London, UK

Series Foreword

Imaging has become pivotal in all aspects of the management of patients with cancer. At the same time it is acknowledged that optimal patient care is best achieved by a multidisciplinary team approach. The explosion of technological developments in imaging over the past years has meant that all members of the multidisciplinary team should understand the potential applications, limitations and advantages of all the evolving and exciting imaging techniques. Equally, to understand the significance of the imaging findings and to contribute actively to management decisions and to the development of new clinical applications for imaging, it is critical that the radiologist should have sufficient background knowledge of different tumours. Thus the radiologist should understand the pathology, the clinical background, the therapeutic options and prognostic indicators of malignancy.

Contemporary Issues in Cancer Imaging — A Multidisciplinary Approach aims to meet the growing requirement for radiologists to have detailed knowledge of the individual tumours in which they are involved in making management decisions. A series of single subject issues, each of which will be dedicated to a single tumour site, edited by recognized expert guest editors, will include contributions from basic scientists, pathologists, surgeons, oncologists, radiologists and others.

While the series is written predominantly for the radiologist, it is hoped that individual issues will contain sufficient varied information to be of interest to all medical disciplines and to other health professionals managing patients with cancer. As with imaging, advances have occurred in all these disciplines related to cancer management and it is our fervent hope that this series, bringing together expertise from such a range of related specialities, will not only promote the understanding and rational application of modern imaging but will also help to achieve the ultimate goal of improving outcomes of patients with cancer.

Rodney Reznek
London

Janet Husband
London

Introduction

In the United Kingdom well over 30,000 new cases of lung cancer are diagnosed each year and there are a roughly similar number of deaths attibutable to the disease annually. In recent years there has been a paradigm shift in emphasis in the management of patients with lung cancer: a 'team approach' is now considered most appropriate and most institutions now have dedicated groups of multidisciplinary specialists who contribute to clinical management. This multidisciplinary approach is reflected in the present volume dedicated to lung cancer. Individual chapters focus on the clinical aspects, pathology, radiology (including screening, diagnosis of symptomatic cases and staging) and treatment options in lung cancer. Because of the recent interest in the potential role of positron emission tomography for a variety of malignancies, a separate chapter is devoted to this technique. Whilst the volume is primarily directed at radiologists, it is hoped that the volume will also be of value to other medical specialists who regularly manage patients with lung cancer.

Sujal R. Desai

Clinical Considerations in Lung Cancer

Pallav Shah

Royal Brompton Hospital, London, UK

Introduction

Lung cancer remains one of the commonest malignancies, accounting for 20% of all cancers in men with a lifetime risk of 1 in 13 and 12% of all cancers in women with a lifetime risk of 1 in 23 [1]. In the United Kingdom roughly 40,000 new cases are recorded each year. The estimated incidence for lung cancer in males in 2005 in the United States was 92,305 with approximately 91,537 males expected to die from the disease [2]. The risk of lung cancer is about fourfold greater in men than in women and this increases with age: in the European Union the incidence of lung cancer is 7 per 100,000 for men and 3 per 100,000 for women at the age of 35 years, but in patients aged over 75, the rates are 440 and 72 in men and women respectively [3]. Wide geographical variations in the incidence of lung cancer are also reported and this is primarily related to worldwide variations in smoking behaviour.

Aetiology

Smoking cigarettes is far and away the dominant risk factor in patients with lung cancer, accounting for 90% of lung cancers in men and almost 80% of cases in women. The relationship between smoking and lung cancer mortality was first established by Doll and Hill [4]. In their study, newly admitted patients with suspected lung, liver or bowel cancers were questioned. The results demonstrated conclusively that patients with a final diagnosis of lung cancer were more likely to be smokers than those without a final diagnosis of lung cancer. The critical study was a prospective study from a cohort of doctors on the medical register who were recruited via a letter in the *British Medical Journal*; there were 40,000 respondents. Over the subsequent two and half years there were 789 patient deaths, 36 of whom had lung cancer. Doll and Hill found a significant increase in the risk of lung cancer with tobacco consumption [5]. A recent update has also published the 50-year results of this landmark investigation [6].

Occupational asbestos exposure has also been shown to increase the risk of lung cancer, particularly with amphibolic froms of asbestos [7]. The effect is significantly increased in individuals who smoke (up to 16-fold) [8]. Radon, which is a decay product of uranium 238 and radon 226, can also accumulate in homes and some studies have demonstrated an increased risk of lung cancer [9]. Exposure to the following carcinogens has also been associated with an increased risk from lung cancer: arsenic, beryllium, bis-choromethyl ether, cadmium, chromium, nickel, polycyclic aromatic hydrocarbons and vinyl chloride. Consequently, a greater incidence of lung cancer has been observed in industries such as coal-gas, metal refining and smelting processes.

Natural History

Assuming the hypothesis that lung cancer grows from a single cell, it usually takes approximately 40 volume-doublings for the tumour to reach a diameter of 10 cm, which is the average size of the tumour at death (Table 1.1) [10]. The average size at which tumours are diagnosed is 3 cm and they have usually undergone 33 volume doublings. Small cell cancers are the most rapidly dividing cancers and double in volume approximately every 29 days. Thus, small cell cancers have been present, on average, for about 2 years 4 months before becoming detectable. In contrast, adenocarcinomas of the lung are slow growing, doubling in volume every 161 days. Squamous cell carcinomas and poorly differentiated carcinomas tend to be somewhere in between, doubling in volume every 88 days.

Table 1.1. Natural history of untreated lung cancer (adapted from Geddes, 1979 [10])

Cell type	Volume doubling time (days)	Time from malignant change (in years)		
		Earliest diagnosis	Usual diagnosis	death
	Tumour size	1 cm	3 cm	10 cm
Small cell	29	2.4	2.8	3.2
Poorly differentiated	86	7.1	8.2	9.4
Squamous	88	7.1	8.4	9.6
Adenocarcinoma	161	13.2	15.4	17.6

The growth rate of lung cancer also illustrates (Table 1.1) that the disease is usually diagnosed late in its natural history. Against this, it is noteworthy that most tumours are capable of metastasizing after about 20 volume doublings but not detectable until after 30 volume doublings. Hence the majority of patients have advanced disease by the time of presentation.

Clinical Features

Symptoms and Signs due to Local Disease

The majority of patients who are diagnosed with lung cancer have symptoms at presentation [11]. The most common symptoms are chronic cough with or without sputum production (Table 1.2). Excessive sputum production is an occasional feature of bronchoalveolar cell carcinoma. Haemoptysis is a symptom that frequently prompts patients to seek medical attention and is a presenting feature in up to 50% of cases. Chest pain is a common feature and may vary from dull vague pain on the side of the tumour or more severe pain due to chest wall or mediastinal invasion. Local invasion of adjacent structures such as ribs and vertebral bodies by the tumour may also cause severe persistent pain.

Table 1.2. Clinical features of lung cancer

Local disease	Intra-thoracic spread
Symptoms	*Symptoms*
Cough	Chest wall pain
Productive sputum	Shoulder tip pain
Haemoptysis	Weakness in the hand
Chest pain	Hoarse voice
Weight loss	Headaches
	Facial swelling
Clinical signs	
Clubbing of finger nails	*Clinical signs*
Monophonic wheeze	Dilated neck veins
Focal wheezing	Facial plethora
Stridor	Horner's syndrome
	Wasting of the small muscles of the hand

Recurrent focal pneumonia and segmental pneumonia should raise the possibility of an obstructive lesion in the airways and should prompt further investigation. Unilateral and monophonic wheezes are less common features of an obstructive bronchial tumour. Stridor may occur where there is tracheal involvement.

Symptoms and Signs due to Intra-thoracic Extension

Extension of lung cancer to adjacent structures may also lead to clinical symptoms and signs. Breathlessness and chest pain may be caused by pleural involvement or pericardial involvement. The subsequent pleural or pericardial effusions may cause breathlessness, and in the case of pericardial involvement may also lead to cardiovascular compromise.

Right upper lobe tumours or adjacent mediastinal nodes may invade or externally compress the superior vena cava (SVC). Such patients then present with a relatively classical SVC syndrome comprising headaches, facial fullness or plethora and oedema with congested neck and chest veins. The SVC syndrome is a presenting feature in about 10% of patients with small cell lung cancer. Apical tumours may also extend to involve the superior sympathetic chain leading to a Horner's syndrome, and brachial plexus involvement causes shoulder and neck pain with atrophy of the small muscles of the hand. Left-sided tumours may compress the recurrent laryngeal nerve as it courses above the aortic arch leading to a hoarse voice and left vocal cord paralysis. Direct tumour invasion or enlarged mediastinal nodes may cause oesophageal compression and hence dysphagia.

Symptoms and Signs due to Distant Spread

Weight loss is a relative common complaint in patients with lung cancer, which is usually associated with a poor outcome; indeed a decrease of weight exceeding 20% of baseline body weight, in the preceding month, is often indicative of metastatic disease. Patients with liver metastases often present with weight loss. Lung cancer also frequently spreads to the adrenal glands, bone, brain and skin. Involvement of these sites may cause localized pain. Bone metastases can occur at any site but tend to occur in the ribs, vertebrae, humeral and femoral bones. With brain metastases there may also be neurological symptoms, such as confusion, personality changes and epileptic seizures. Supraclavicular and anterior cervical lymph nodes may be involved in up to 25% of patients and should be routinely assessed in the evaluation of patients with lung cancer.

Symptoms and Signs due to Para-neoplastic Syndromes

Para-neoplastic syndromes are present in 10–20% of patients with lung cancers. Some of the typical syndromes are displayed in Table 1.3 and are usually due to the ectopic production of hormones or peptides. These patients can present with vague symptoms such as tiredness, nausea, abdominal pain or confusion, or more specific symptoms such as galactorrhoea. Ectopic hormone production is more common in small cell lung cancer and some of the cells show neuro-endocrine characteristics.

Table 1.3. Paraneoplastic syndromes

Common		Rare
General	*General*	
Anorexia,	Fever	Hypercalcitoninemia
Cachexia	Marantic endocarditis	Hypoglycemia
Weight loss		Hypophosphatemia
Clubbing of finger nails	*Connective Tissue/vasculitis*	Lactic acidosis
HPOA	Dermatomyositis/Polymyositis	
	Systemic Lupus Erythematosus	*Haematological*
Endocrine		Amyloidosis
Hypercalcemia	*Cutaneous*	Eosinophilia
SIADH	Acanthosis nigricans	Leucocytosis
	Acquired ichthyosis	Leukoerythroblastic reaction
Haematological	Acquired palmoplantar keratoderma	Polycythemia
Anaemia	Dermatomyositis	Thrombocytopenia
Polycythemia	Erythema annulare	
	Exfoliative dermatitis	*Neurological*
Neurological	Pemphigus	Autonomic neuropathy
Lambert-Eaton	Pruritis	Cerebellar degeneration
myasthenia syndrome		Limbic encephalitis
Peripheral neuropathy	*Endocrine*	Pontine myelinosis
	Acromegaly	Retinopathy
	Carcinoid Syndrome	
	Cushings Syndrome	*Renal*
	Gynaecomastia	Glomeronephritis
		Tubulointerstitial

Key:
HPOA is hypertrophic pulmonary osteo-arthropathy.
SIADH is syndrome of inappropriate antidiuretic hormone secretion.

The range of peptides secreted includes adrenocorticotrophic hormone (ACTH), antidiuretic hormone (ADH), calcitonin, oxytocin and parathyroid hormone. Although elevated levels of these peptides are found in patients with lung cancer only about 5% of patients develop the clinical syndromes. Digital clubbing with hypertrophic pulmonary osteo-arthropathy (HPOA) is considered a non-metastatic manifestation of lung cancer. Peripheral neuropathy and neurological syndromes such as Lambert-Eaton myasthenic syndrome may also be associated with lung cancer.

Diagnosis of Lung Cancer

Histopathological and cytological confirmation of the diagnosis is an essential step in the management of patients with lung cancer. Diagnosis and staging can be approached together to provide better prognostic information and more appropriately planned treatment. A computed tomography (CT) scan of the thorax and abdomen should be the initial diagnostic test after chest radiography (Fig. 1.1). The CT study will not only provide information about the location of the primary lesion but also about possible involvement of adjacent structures and provisional staging information (note that the issue of the imaging diagnosis and staging of lung cancer are the subjects of separate chapters in this volume). In addition to CT scanning, many patients with suspected lung cancer will be referred for fibreoptic bronchoscopy. This is discussed in the following section.

Fibroptic Bronchoscopy

Bronchoscopy is one of the key investigations in the assessment of patients with suspected lung cancer since the procedure not only permits visual examination of the major airways down to subsegmental level, but also provides a variety of methods of sampling abnormal tissue for cytological or histopathological diagnosis. Central tumours vary in appearance from extrinsic polypoid lesions through diffuse plaque-like infiltrations to subtle mucosal irregularity (Fig. 1.2). Large tumour masses and enlarged lymph nodes may also cause extrinsic narrowing of the airways.

   With central lesions, a number of sampling techniques such as bronchial washings, bronchial biopsy and bronchial brushings may be utilized. With washings,

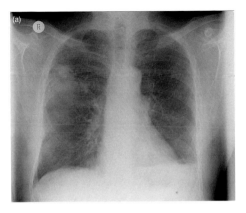
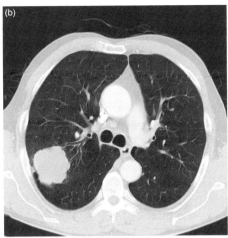

Figure 1.1 (a) Chest radiograph and (b) CT scan demonstrating a right upper lobe mass

approximately 20 ml of saline is instilled around the area of abnormality and the aspirate sent for cytological analysis. Bronchial biopsy is the most useful test for polypoid lesions. Forceps can be inserted through the instrument channel of the bronchoscope to pinch biopsies of the lesion under direct vision. A cytological brush can also be used to scrape some cells from the abnormal area. A combination of these techniques should provide a spot-on diagnosis in up to 90% of patients where the lesion is located in the larger central airways [12].

Where the lesion is peripheral, techniques such as segmental lavage, selective brushings and fluoroscopic transbronchial fine needle aspiration may be utilized. However, the yield is usually lower at around 40% [13, 14]. Hence, CT guided biopsy is the usual technique for obtaining a diagnosis in peripherally located lesions. New techniques have been developed which facilitate bronchoscopic sampling of peripheral lesions including magnetic navigation guided bronchoscopy. A spiral CT with 1.5–3 mm slice thickness is required and specific landmarks marked at virtual bronchoscopy. A catheter with a magnetic tracking device is then inserted through the instrument channel (Super Dimensions Bronchus^{TM}) and the catheter tip is positioned at the same landmarks and calibrated with the CT scan. This allows the CT data to be overlayed on the patient and the system can then be used to guide the catheter with the magnetic tracking device to the target lesion. Once the target is reached, the tracking device is removed, the biopsy forceps or

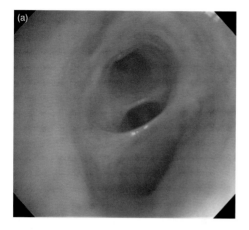
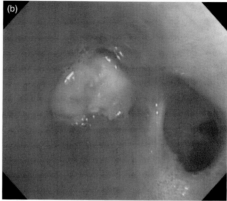
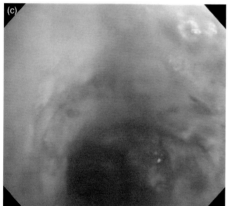

Figure 1.2 Videobronchoscopy appearance of: (a) normal endobronchial airway at segmental level (b) polypoid exophytic tumour; (c) submucosal lesion (for a colour version of this figure please see the colour plate section)

needle is inserted through the catheter and appropriate samples obtained for diagnosis.

Transbronchial fine needle aspiration (TBNA) is a technique that is being incorporated into the routine clinical assessment of patients with suspected lung cancer [15, 16]. It enables sampling of mediastinal and hilar lymph nodes and provides both diagnostic and staging information. The procedure should be planned according to data provided by a recent CT study. The TBNA needle is inserted through the bronchoscopic channel then inserted at the appropriate point through the airway (Fig. 1.3). The needle is pushed all the way through and suction is applied to the other end with a 20 ml syringe. A jabbing action during the procedure allows cytological material to be aspirated into the needle. The sample obtained is then spread on slides or injected into a liquid media and

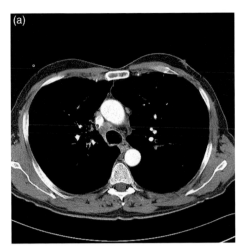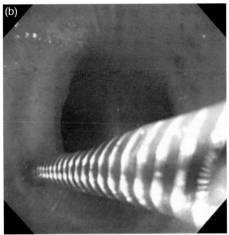

Figure 1.3 (a) CT scan of a patient with right upper lobe tumour and enlarged right paratracheal lymph node and (b) videobronchoscopy appearance of the trachea demonstrating transbronchial fine needle aspiration of the right paratracheal lymph node (for a colour version of this figure please see the colour plate section)

sent for cytological analysis. TBNA should be performed before inspection of the airways so as not to contaminate the samples and minimize the risk of false positive results. This is important as TBNA in this context provides both diagnostic and staging information. On site cytological analysis appears to enhance the diagnostic yield of TBNA and reduces the number of samples that have to be obtained for diagnosis [17]. It must be remembered that TBNA results do not exclude neoplastic disease and should be followed up by further investigations, such as mediastinoscopy, in appropriate cases. TBNA is a safe and effective technique. Complications are rare and consist of pneumothorax, pneumomediastinum and bleeding [15, 16].

Puncture bronchoscopes have been developed which integrate video bronchoscopes with a linear array ultrasound probe to improve the diagnostic yield from TBNA. This integrated bronchoscope can be used to assess the mediastinum accurately, which significantly improves the diagnosis and staging of patients with suspected lung cancer. The bronchoscope has a dedicated needle, which can be inserted through the instrument channel of the bronchoscope so TBNA can be performed with real time ultrasound imaging. A preliminary study in 70 patients has demonstrated a high sensitivity (95.7%) and accuracy (97.1%) in patients with suspected malignancy [18].

Prognosis

The three main prognostic factors for bronchogenic carcinoma are cell type, disease staging or extent and treatment modality. Small cell lung cancer carries the worst prognosis and untreated median survival is only around three months. With chemotherapy this improves to around nine months. In contrast, survival of non-small cell lung cancer is better. Disease stage strongly influences treatment and survival. Patients with Stage I disease who are amenable to surgery have a five-year survival rate – over 60% – whereas patients with stage III or IV disease who are only amenable to palliative treatment have a five-year survival rate of less than 10%. The EUROCARE data demonstrate marked variations in survival between European countries [19]. For example, one-year and five-year survival rates in Finland were 43% and 16%, respectively, compared to 23% and 6% in the United Kingdom. Other prognostic factors are age. The EUROCARE data demonstrate a poorer prognosis with increasing age [19]. This relationship is maintained with cell type and disease stage.

Summary

Smoking is the main aetiological factor in the pathogenesis of lung cancer. Despite this knowledge, the incidence and mortality for lung cancer remains high. Symptoms occur late in the natural history of lung cancer and hence the majority of lung cancers present late with advanced disease. Accurate diagnosis and staging are an essential guide to treatment and prognosis.

REFERENCES

1. Quinn, M., Babb, P., Brock, A., Kibly, L., Jones, J. (2001). *Cancer Trends in England & Wales 1950–1999*. London: Office for National Statistics.
2. Stat Bite (2005). US death rates for selected cancers in men, 1969–2002. *J Natl Cancer Inst.*, **97**(18), 1328.
3. Ferley, J., Bjalk, R. J., Pisani, P., *et al.* (1996). Eucan90: Cancer in the European Union. *IARC Cancer base ND 1*. lyon: IARc.
4. Doll, R., Hill, A. B. (1950). Smoking and cancer of the lung; preliminary report. *Br Med J*, **2**, 739.
5. Doll, R., Hill, A. B. (1954). The mortality of doctors in relation to their smoking habits. A preliminary report. *Br Med J*, **4877**, 1451.

6. Doll, R., Peto, R., Boreham, J., Sutherland, I. (2004). Mortality in relation to smoking: 50 years' observations on male British doctors. *BMJ*, **328**, 1519–28.

7. Warnock, M. L., Isenberg, W. (1986). Asbestos burden and the pathology of lung cancer. *Chest*, **89**, 20–6.

8. Hammond, E. C., Selikoff, I. J., Seidman, H. (1979). Asbestos exposure, cigarette smoking and death rates. *Ann N Y Acad Sci*, **330**, 473–90.

9. Lubin, J. H., Boice, J. D. Jr (1997). Lung cancer risk from residential radon: meta-analysis of eight epidemiologic studies. *J Natl Cancer Inst*, **89**, 49–57.

10. Geddes, D. M. (1979). The natural history of lung cancer: a review based on rates of tumour growth. *Br J Dis Chest*, **73**, 1–17.

11. Yang, P., Allen, M. S., Aubry, M. C., Wampfler, J. A., Marks, R. S., Edell, E. S., *et al.* (2005). Clinical features of 5,628 primary lung cancer patients: experience at mayo clinic from 1997 to 2003. *Chest*, **128**, 452–62.

12. Schreiber, G., McCrory, D. C. (2003). Performance characteristics of different modalities for diagnosis of suspected lung cancer: summary of published evidence. *Chest*, **123**(1 Suppl), 115S–28S.

13. Lam, W. K., So, S.Y., Hsu, C., *et al.* (1983). Fibreoptic bronchoscopy in the diagnosis of bronchial cancer: comparison of washings, brushings and biopsies in central and peripheral tumours. *Clin Oncol*, **9**, 35–42.

14. Reichenberger, F., Weber, J., Tamm, M., Bolliger, C. T., Dalquen, P., Perruchoud, A. P., Soler, M. (1999). The value of transbronchial needle aspiration in the diagnosis of peripheral pulmonary lesions. *Chest*, **116**, 704–8.

15. Harrow, E. M., Abi-Saleh, W., Blum, J., *et al.* (2000). The utility of transbronchial needle aspiration in the staging of bronchogenic carcinoma. *Am J Respir Crit Care Med*, **161**(2Pt1), 601–7.

16. Shah, P. L., Singh, S., Bower, M., Livini, N., Padley, S., Nicholson, A. G. (in press). The role of transbronchial fine needle aspiration (TBNA) in an integrated care pathway for the assessment of patients with suspected lung cancer. *J Thor Oncol*.

17. Davenport, R. D. (1990). Rapid on-site evaluation of transbronchial aspirates. *Chest*, **98**, 59–61.

18. Yasufuku, K., Chiyo, M., Sekine, Y., Chhajed, P. N., Shibuya, K., Iizasa, T., Fujisawa, T. (2004). Real-time endobronchial ultrasound-guided transbronchial needle aspiration of mediastinal and hilar lymph nodes. *Chest*, **126**, 122–8.

19. Janssen-Heijnen, M. L. G., Coebergh, J. W. (2003). The changing epidemiology of lung cancer in Europe. *Lung Cancer*, **41**, 245–58.

2

Pathology of Lung Cancer

Sabine Pomplun

Department of Histopathology, King's College Hospital, London, UK

Introduction

Lung cancer remains one of the most common cancers, accounting for 12.6% of all new cancers and just under 20% of all cancer deaths. It is widely accepted that the incidence of lung cancer is closely associated with population-related smoking behaviour [1, 2]; the relative risk for smokers, as compared to non-smokers, is of the order of 8–15-fold for men and 3–10-fold for women dependent on factors such as the average cigarette consumption, duration of smoking, age at which the subject starts or the time since quitting, type of tobacco and the pattern of inhalation [3].

Traditionally, squamous cell carcinoma has the strongest association with tobacco smoking, followed by small cell carcinoma and adenocarcinoma. However, the association with adenocarcinoma has become stronger over time and this histological subtype has become the most common type in many western countries. There are also recognized occupational exposures to carcinogens known to be associated with lung cancer, the most important being asbestos, crystalline silica, radon, mixtures of polycyclic aromatic hydrocarbons and heavy metals. Welding and painting are consistently associated with an increased risk of lung cancer, but the causative agents are still unknown [3].

Almost all lung malignancies are carcinomas with other histological types accounting for less than 1%. In a published series on cancer incidence [4], small cell carcinomas comprised approximately 20% of cases and large cell carcinoma around 9%. The remainder are squamous cell carcinomas and adenocarcinomas, with the former being more common in men and the latter more prevalent in women.

Genetic and Molecular Alterations in Lung Cancer

The multistep carcinogenesis theory can be applied to development of lung cancer. However, no sequential genetic alterations have yet been established since lung cancers are genetically diverse. Many environmental carcinogens present in tobacco smoke or industrial pollutants can act as initiators to help the cells acquire genetic alterations that will give a growth advantage. Progression occurs with the accumulation of genetic changes, which include allelic loss, chromosomal instability and imbalance, mutations in oncogenes and tumour suppressor genes and aberrant expression of genes [5–9]. Although some genetic changes (i.e. p53 mutations, inactivation of retinoblastoma gene and LOH 3p), occur in all tumour types, their frequency and time of occurrence differ in small cell and non-small cell lung cancer. Variations have also been identified between squamous cell carcinomas and adenocarcinomas [10].

The association with EGFR-overexpression in squamous cell carcinomas is the subject of research and development of new therapeutic strategies [11].

Pre-invasive Lesions

Squamous dysplasia (Fig. 2.1) and carcinoma in situ are defined as precursor abnormalities for squamous cell carcinoma that may occur as single or multifocal lesions existing either as foci of isolated disease or accompany invasive carcinoma. Although the multistage model of squamous cell carcinoma following the steps of hyperplasia, metaplasia, dysplasia, carcinoma in situ and invasive carcinoma is accepted [12, 13], there are, at present, no data to support the notion that the progression to invasive carcinoma can be predicted from evaluation of the degree of dysplasia. This notwithstanding, it is generally believed that high-grade dysplasia carries a greater risk of being associated with invasive tumour. It is important to appreciate that foci of squamous dysplasia cannot be detected by conventional imaging techniques but may be identified at bronchoscopy.

Another lesion worthy of mentioning is that of atypical adenomatoid hyperplasia (AAH). In this entity, there is a localized peripheral lesion (usually measuring less than 5 mm in diameter), characterized by proliferation of atypical cells lining the alveoli generally in the absence of underlying interstitial inflammation and fibrosis (Fig. 2.2). Most foci of AAH have been identified incidentally in resection specimens for carcinoma, particularly in patients with adenocarcinoma. Radiological

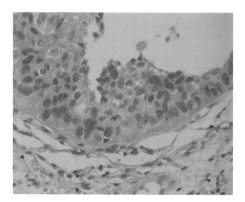

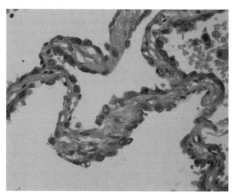

Figure 2.1 Squamous cell dysplasia with no invasion of basement membrane (H&E, 40x) (for a colour version of this figure please see the colour plate section)

Figure 2.2 Atypical adenomatous hyperplasia. Atypical pneumocytes lining alveolar walls with no associated fibrosis or inflammatory infiltrate (H&E, 40x) (for a colour version of this figure please see the colour plate section)

experience of AAH is restricted to screening studies with CT [14, 15] and typical lesions of AAH present as small non-solid nodules of ground-glass attenuation, generally not visualized on plain chest radiography. Although AAH is widely believed to be a pre-malignant condition, there is, at present, no indication for surgical or medical therapy in patients without cancer, other than follow-up. To date there are no differences in post-operative survival of cancer patients with or without AAH [16–19]. Like AAH, another rare lesion which is thought to have malignant potential is diffuse idiopathic pulmonary neuroendocrine cell hyperplasia (DIPNECH) [20, 21].

Common Histological Subtypes of Lung Cancer

Lung cancers frequently show histological heterogeneity with variation in appearance and differentiation [22] and this fact can prove problematic for classification purposes, especially when interpreting small biopsies.

The following classification is based on the World Health Organisation classification of lung tumours [23] and divides tumour groups according to their most common location on CT; this classification has some logic since there is an association between the tumour location and the histological subtype. The radiological features of lung cancer are covered in greater detail elsewhere in this issue. However, a brief discussion of the imaging findings is pertinent in the present chapter.

Centrally Located Tumours (Tumours Associated with Main Stem, Lobar or Segmental Bronchi)

Squamous Cell Carcinoma (SCC)

The majority of SCC present as hilar, perihilar or mediastinal masses with or without lung collapse and mediastinal shift [24]; SCC is the most common cell type to show cavitation. Peripheral SCC also occurs, presenting either as a nodule or a larger mass [25]. On macroscopic examination, the tumours are typically white or grey in colour. A centrally located tumour may obstruct the bronchial lumen resulting in greater or lesser degrees of atelectasis, stasis of bronchial secretion, lipoid pneumonia or infective bronchopneumonia in the more distal lung. More advanced disease may directly involve hilar lymph nodes, the pleura, chest wall and mediastinal structures. Metastases from squamous carcinoma occur most commonly in the brain, liver, adrenal glands, gastro-intestinal tract and lymph nodes. Bone metastases are also frequent and typically osteolytic.

Histologically, SCC is defined as a malignant epithelial tumour showing keratinisation (Fig. 2.3) and/or intercellular bridges (Fig. 2.4). Four variants of SCC (papillary, clear cell, basaloid and a small cell variant) are recognized based mainly on the varying degrees of differentiation. On immunohistochemical examination, most SCCs express high-molecular keratins (34-beta E12, CK5/6) and carcinogenic embryonic antigen (CEA), but very few express thyroid transcription factor-1 (TTF-1) [26−29].

Whilst disease stage and performance status at presentation are the dominant predictors for survival in patients with lung cancer, the degree of histological differentiation may also have an independent bearing on outcome. Whereas well-differentiated SCC tends to be locally aggressive, poorly differentiated tumours have a tendency to metastasize at an earlier stage to distant sites [25]. Furthermore, because of the pattern of direct tumour extension (mainly due to subepithelial growth or carcinoma in situ), SCC has a high propensity for local recurrence [30].

Small Cell Lung Cancer (SCLC)

SCLC typically presents as a central (hilar or perihilar) mass with or without associated lobar collapse but commonly with extensive mediastinal lymph node enlargement and superior vena cava obstruction. Peripheral SCLC (which accounts for approximately 5% of cases) are also recognized but are radiologically indistinguishable from other peripheral cancers [31]. Macroscopically, SCLC is white-tan

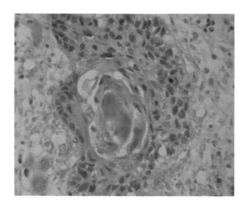

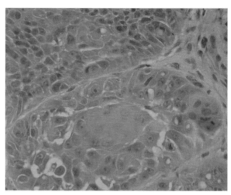

Figure 2.3 Squamous cell carcinoma showing keratin pearl (H&E, 40x) (for a colour version of this figure please see the colour plate section)

Figure 2.4 Squamous cell carcinoma with intercellular bridges (H&E, 40x) (for a colour version of this figure please see the colour plate section)

in colour, generally soft and friable with visible areas of necrosis. At microscopy, SCLC is defined as a malignant epithelial tumour composed of small cells with scant cytoplasm, indistinct cell borders, finely granular nuclear chromatin, absent nucleoli showing nuclear moulding. Necrosis is usually a prominent feature and evidence of mitotic activity is usually high (Fig. 2.5).

Combined small cell carcinoma is a small cell component seen together with any non-small cell cancer, most commonly adenocarcinoma, squamous cell carcinoma or large cell carcinoma [21, 32]. Direct tumour spread is often seen as submucosal extension and intralymphatic spread. On immunohistochemical evaluation, the tumour can be seen to express keratins (Fig. 2.6) and neuroendocrine makers including CD56, chromogranin and synaptophysin. Up to 90% of SCLC are also positive for TTF-1 [33, 34]. The exact cell of origin of SCLC remains unknown. There is emerging genetic evidence that small cell carcinoma shows more similarities with large cell neuroendocrine carcinoma than with either typical or atypical carcinoid.

Peripherally Located Tumours (Usually No Association with the Bronchial Tree) (Fig. 2.7)

Adenocarcinomas

Most adenocarcinomas present as peripheral nodules measuring less than 4 cm in diameter. On CT, 'solid' nodules, ground-glass opacities and combined solid/-ground-glass opacities are all recognized patterns. The more extensive the solid

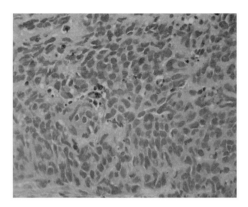

Figure 2.5 Small cell carcinoma, note the high apoptosis rate and the absence of nucleoli (H&E, 40x) (for a colour version of this figure please see the colour plate section)

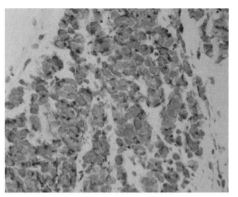

Figure 2.6   Keratin stain in small cell carcinoma with characteristic perinuclear dot-positivity (MNF116, 40x) (for a colour version of this figure please see the colour plate section)

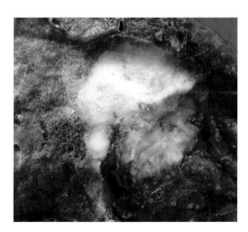

Figure 2.7 Macroscopic picture of peripheral lung cancer (*image courtesy of Professor Andrew G. Nicholson, Royal Brompton Hospital, London*) (for a colour version of this figure please see the colour plate section)

component of the lesion, the greater the likelihood for invasive growth and thus, a less favourable prognosis. Several macroscopic patterns are recognized. A solid peripheral nodule is by far the most common [35], but central or endobronchial tumours also occur. Diffuse pneumonia-like lobar consolidation is often seen with bronchoalveolar cell carcinomas (BAC). Diffuse bilateral lung disease also occurs with multiple nodules ranging in size from large to tiny. Such an appearance may need to be differentiated from metastatic disease. Adenocarcinomas can preferentially invade and disseminate along the pleura thus mimicking the features of malignant pleural mesothelioma [36]. Macroscopically, adenocarcinoma of the

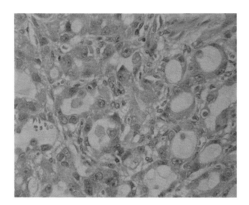

Figure 2.8 Acinar pattern of adenocarcinoma (H&E, 40x) (for a colour version of this figure please see the colour plate section)

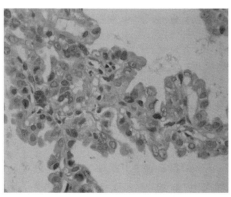

Figure 2.9   Non-mucinous bronchio-alveolar carcinoma, alveoli lined with atypical cells showing papillary infoldings (H&E, 40x) (for a colour version of this figure please see the colour plate section)

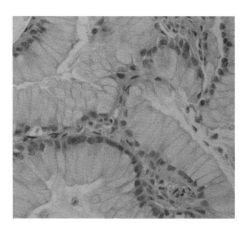

Figure 2.10 Mucinous bronchiolo-alveolar carcinoma with high-columnar lining cells (H&E, 40x) (for a colour version of this figure please see the colour plate section)

lung appears as a grey-white coloured lesion, often with central fibrosis which puckers the pleural surface and can show necrosis; cavitation is a rare feature.

Histologically, adenocarcinoma is defined as a malignant epithelial tumour showing glandular differentiation or mucin production with acinar (Fig. 2.8), papillary, bronchoalveolar cell or solid with mucinous growth patterns or indeed a mixture of these. Most tumours show a variety of growth patterns (mixed subtype) and 'pure' BACs are less common, but do have a more favourable outcome when localized. BACs have been divided into non-mucinous (Fig. 2.9), mucinous (Fig. 2.10) and mixed types, all of which represent well- or

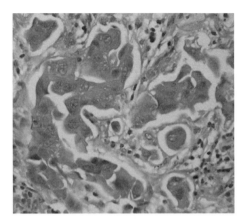

Figure 2.11 Micropapillary pattern of adenocarcinoma ('inside-out glands'), associated with poorer outcome (H&E, 40x) (for a colour version of this figure please see the colour plate section)

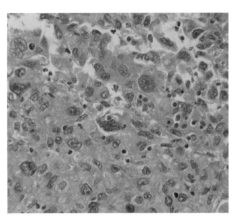

Figure 2.12 Large cell carcinoma. Large polygonal cells with prominent nucleoli, no squamous and no glandular differentiation (H&E, 40x) (for a colour version of this figure please see the colour plate section)

moderately- differentiated tumours. The pathologist should make a careful search for an invasive component (particularly if there was a solid area on imaging), since this may have prognostic significance. Acinar, papillary and solid tumours can show high, moderate or poor differentiation, depending on the severity of cytological atypia and the degree of mucin production [21]. As might be expected, poorly differentiated tumours tend to show more frequent local recurrence and lymph node metastases than well-differentiated tumours [37]. Papillary or micropapillary growth patterns (Fig. 2.11) are also associated with an unfavourable outcome [38–40].

Large cell carcinoma

Large cell carcinoma is defined as a malignant epithelial neoplasm lacking cytological features of small cell carcinoma and glandular or squamous differentiation (Fig. 2.12). Most tumours are peripheral, with the notable exception of the basaloid form. Large cell carcinomas encompass large cell neuroendocrine carcinoma, basaloid carcinoma, clear cell carcinoma, lymphoepithelioma-like carcinoma and large cell carcinoma with a rhabdoid phenotype; the latter four patterns are rare. Large cell neuroendocrine carcinoma (LCNEC) shows an organoid nested growth pattern occasionally with rosettes suggesting neuroendocrine differentiation. The prominent nucleoli of tumour cells distinguish this tumour from

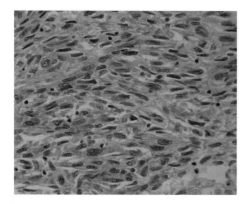

Figure 2.13 Sarcomatoid carcinoma with malignant spindle cells with no squamous or glandular differentiation (H&E, 40x) (for a colour version of this figure please see the colour plate section)

small cell carcinoma. Neuroendocrine differentiation needs to be confirmed with immunohistochemical markers such as chromogranin, synaptophysin and neural-cellular adhesion molecule (NCAM). Around 50% of LCNEC express TTF-1 [41, 42] and like small cell carcinoma, large cell carcinoma can be seen together with other non-small cell types, such as adenocarcinoma, squamous or sarcomatoid carcinoma (so-called, combined large cell carcinomas). Combination with small cell carcinoma also occurs, but such tumours are generally classified as combined small cell carcinomas. At present there is debate about whether the presence of neuroendocrine differentiation has any prognostic or therapeutic implication [43–48].

Adenosquamous Carcinoma

This tumour is defined as a carcinoma showing both squamous and glandular differentiation with each component comprising at least 10% of the tumour. Most tumours are located peripherally and exhibit a central scar. Grading and staging is similar to that of other non-small cell carcinomas, but these tumours appear to have a dismal prognosis, with an overall 5-year survival rate of just over 20% [49].

Sarcomatoid carcinoma is rare, but can present as central or peripheral nodule. This entity encompasses pleomorphic carcinoma, spindle cell carcinoma (Fig. 2.13), giant cell carcinoma, carcinosarcoma and pulmonary blastoma. All these tumours represent malignant epithelial neoplasms that have undergone divergent mesenchymal differentiation [50] and all have a worse prognosis than other non-small cell carcinomas.

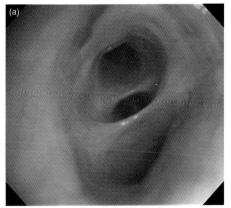

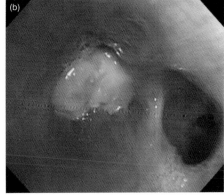

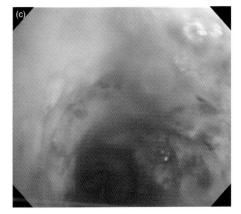

Figure 1.2 Videobronchoscopy appearance of:
(a) Normal endobronchial airway at segmental
level (b) Polypoid exophytic tumour;
(c) submucosal lesion

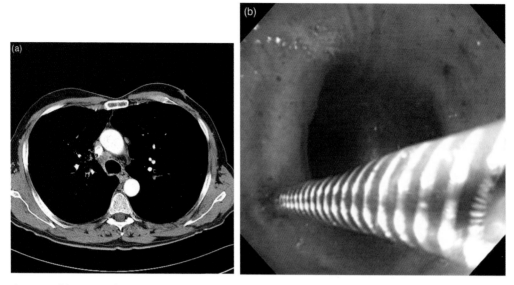

Figure 1.3 (a) CT scan of a patient with right upper lobe tumour and enlarged right paratracheal lymph node and (b) videobronchoscopy appearance of the trachea demonstrating transbronchial fine needle aspiration of the right paratracheal lymph node

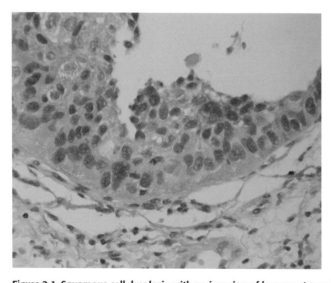

Figure 2.1 Squamous cell dysplasia with no invasion of basement membrane (H&E, 40x)

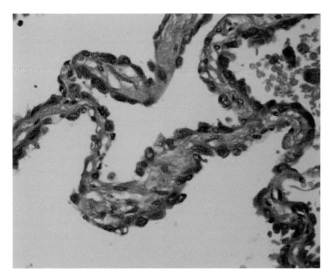

Figure 2.2 Atypical adenomatous hyperplasia. Atypical pneumocytes lining alveolar walls with no associated fibrosis or inflammatory infiltrate (H&E, 40x)

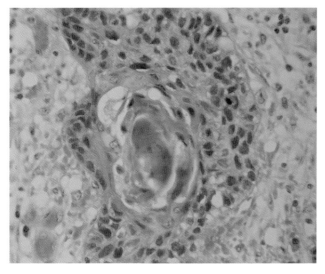

Figure 2.3 Squamous cell carcinoma showing keratin pearl (H&E, 40x)

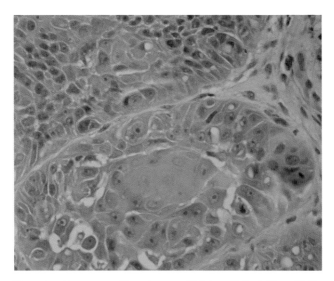

Figure 2.4 Squamous cell carcinoma with intercellular bridges (H&E, 40x)

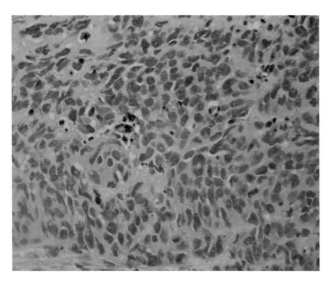

Figure 2.5 Small cell carcinoma, note the high apoptosis rate and the absence of nucleoli (H&E, 40x)

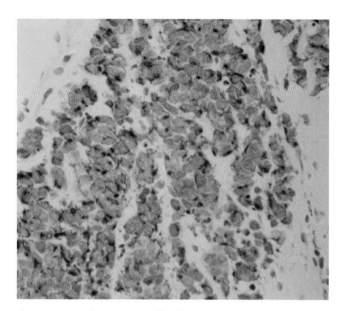

Figure 2.6 Keratin stain in small cell carcinoma with characteristic perinuclear dot-positivity (MNF116, 40x)

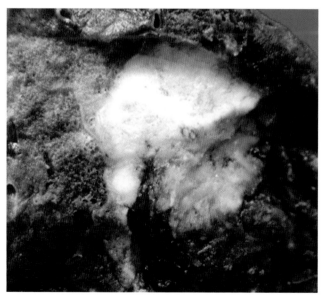

Figure 2.7 Macroscopic picture of peripheral lung cancer (image courtesy of Professor Andrew G. Nicholson, Royal Brompton Hospital, London)

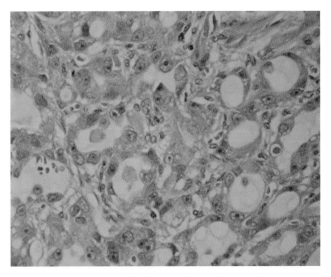

Figure 2.8 Acinar pattern of adenocarcinoma (H&E, 40x)

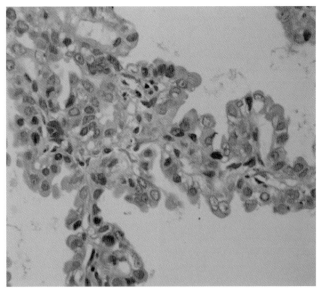

Figure 2.9 Non-mucinous bronchio-alveolar carcinoma, alveoli lined with atypical cells showing papillary infoldings (H&E, 40x)

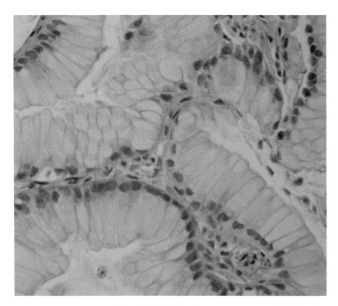

Figure 2.10 Mucinous bronchiolo-alveolar carcinoma with high-columnar lining cells (H&E, 40x)

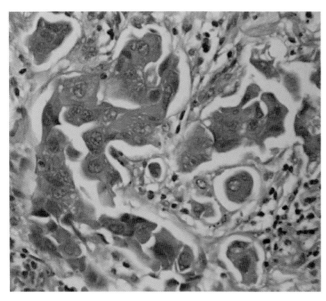

Figure 2.11 Micropapillary pattern of adenocarcinoma ('inside-out glands'),associated with poorer outcome (H&E, 40x)

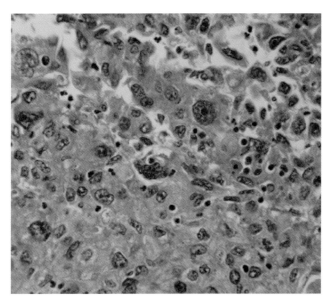

Figure 2.12 Large cell carcinoma. Large polygonal cells with prominent nucleoli, no squamous and no glandular differentiation (H&E, 40x)

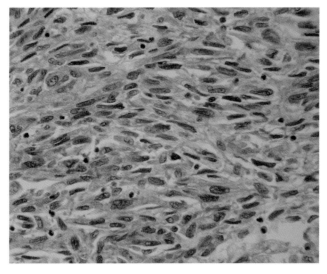

Figure 2.13 Sarcomatoid carcinoma with malignant spindle cells with no squamous or glandular differentiation (H&E, 40x)

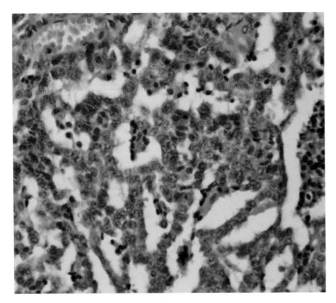

Figure 2.14 Typical carcinoid. Uniform cells with no mitoses and no necrosis(H&E, 40x)

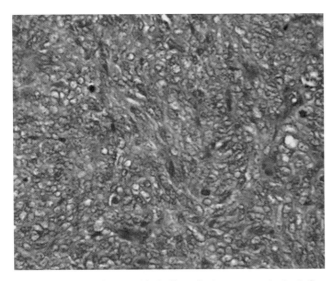

Figure 2.15 Atypical carcinoid, similar cells, but scattered mitotic figures (H&E,40x)

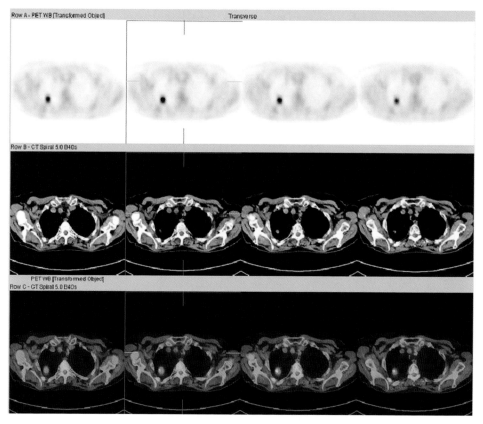

Figure 6.1 A right apical solitary pulmonary nodule. This demonstrates intense ^{18}FDG activity (SUV $=$ 5.6) and was subsequently found to represent a squamous cell carcinoma

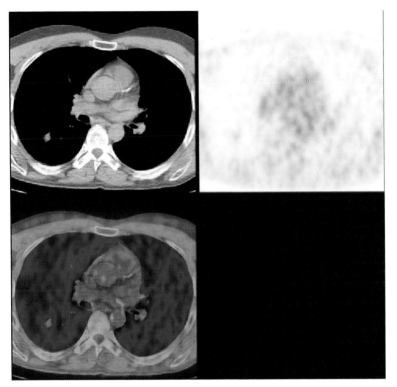

Figure 6.2   A right lower lobe nodule that does not demonstrate [18]FDG activity and is therefore likely to be benign

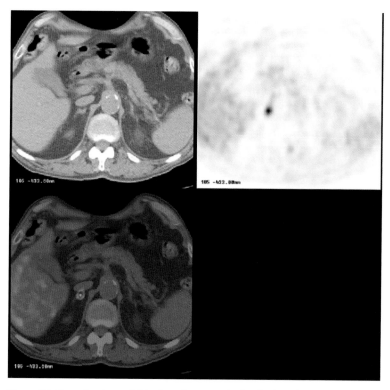

Figure 6.4 A small volume right adrenal metastasis that had not been suspected on the CT appearances but demonstrates abnormal activity on the PET scan

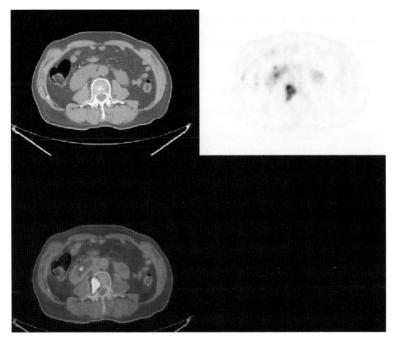

Figure 6.5   A previously undiagnosed vertebral bone metastasis identified by PET but with no abnormality seen on the CT component of the examination

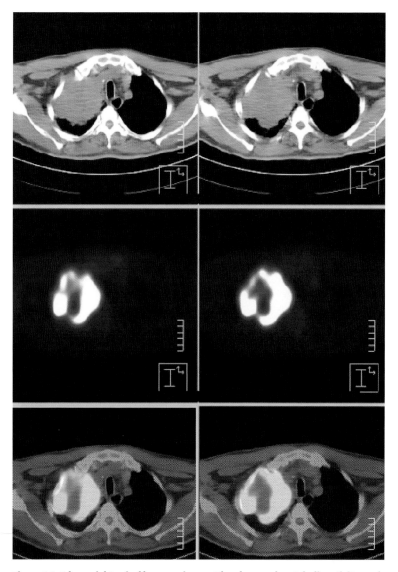

Figure 6.6 A large right apical lung carcinoma. The abnormal metabolic activity can be seen to extend into the chest wall anteriorly on the fused PET/CT images

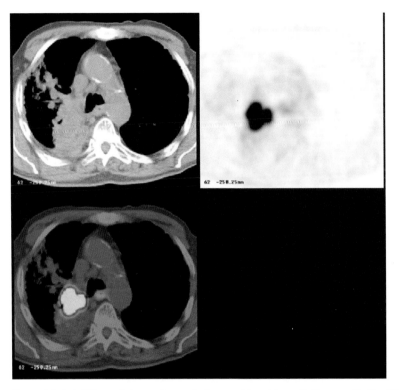

Figure 6.7 A right lower lobe carcinoma being considered for radiotherapy. On the CT it is difficult to determine the true extent of the tumour tissue and how much of the mass is due to benign collapse and consolidation. The PET images clearly show the anatomical boundaries between the benign and malignant tissue

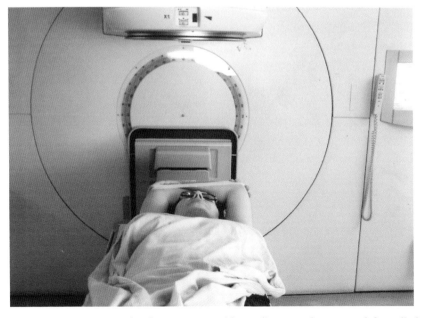

Figure 8.1 Lung cancer patient in treatment position on linear accelerator couch for radiotherapy

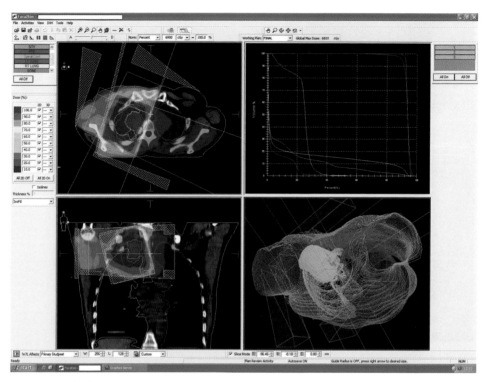

Figure 8.2 Radiotherapy treatment plan for lung tumour. Colour washes indicate percentage isodose to patient target volume

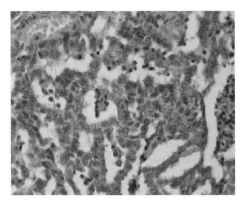

Figure 2.14 Typical carcinoid. Uniform cells with no mitoses and no necrosis (H&E, 40x) (for a colour version of this figure please see the colour plate section)

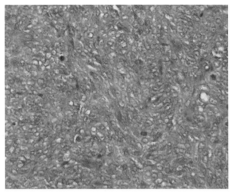

Figure 2.15 Atypical carcinoid, similar cells, but scattered mitotic figures (H&E, 40x) (for a colour version of this figure please see the colour plate section)

Endobronchial Tumours

Carcinoid, Typical and Atypical

Carcinoid tumours are defined as epithelial tumours showing a particular growth pattern (i.e. trabecular, organoid, insular, palisading, ribbon- and rosette-like), which suggests neuroendocrine differentiation. The tumour cells in carcinoid lesions are usually uniform containing small nuclei with a finely granular chromatin pattern and eosinophilic cytoplasm. Carcinoid tumours are conveniently divided into two types: 'typical' carcinoid (in which there are less than 2 mitoses per 10 HPF and no evidence of necrosis) (Fig. 2.14) and 'atypical' carcinoid (containing more than 2 mitoses per 10 HPF and/or foci of necrosis) (Fig. 2.15). Although the common perception is that carcinoid tumours are endobronchial lesions, typical carcinoids may be found at any site in the lungs [51], and atypical carcinoids are more commonly found in the periphery [52]. It is interesting to note that almost half of all carcinoids are incidental findings [53]. Macroscopically, these tumours are firm and tan to yellow in colour, often associated with a bronchus. Histologically, they show a variety of growth patterns (listed above) but in most there is a mixture of these. Carcinoid tumours have traditionally been regarded as benign lesions. However, it must be remembered that between 10% and 15% of typical carcinoids will metastasize to regional lymph nodes at time of presentation and up to 10% may eventually metastasize to distant sites such as liver and bone. Fortunately, even when there are lymph node metastases, typical carcinoid is associated with an excellent prognosis, with 10-year survival rate ranging from 82% to 95% [54]. In stark contrast, atypical carcinoids are not only more frequently associated with metastases at presentation (40–50% in regional lymph nodes and beyond) but also carry a significantly worse 10-year survival of only 35–59% [52]. A tumour size over 3.5 cm, high mitotic rate, pleomorphism and aerogenous spread are recognized adverse prognostic indicators, whereas palisading, papillary formation and pseudoglandular patterns tend to predict a more favourable outcome [52].

Salivary Gland-like Tumours

These comprise mucoepidermoid, adenoid cystic and epithelial-myoepithelial carcinomas. These tumours are rare and usually present with a prominent endobronchial component. There is no documented link with smoking related and, on the whole, follow an indolent course with multiple local recurrences before metastases occur. The only exception perhaps to this general rule, is with high-grade mucoepidermoid carcinoma, which tends to behave similarly to other non-small cell carcinomas. Other much less common tumour types include mesenchymal tumours (i.e. angiosarcomas), pleuro-pulmonary blastomas, melanomas and pulmonary thymomas as well as primary lymphoid malignancies usually present as peripheral masses.

Conclusion

The vast majority of primary lung malignancies are epithelial neoplasms, which demonstrate considerable heterogeneity of morphology and genetic constitution. Tobacco smoking is the single most important risk factor for the development of lung cancer. Histological subtyping, particularly the distinction between small cell and non-small cell carcinomas, is a dominant and independent prognostic indicator. With the identification of different tumour types and their presumably different disease pathways there is hope for the development of new therapeutic strategies.

REFERENCES

1. Gilliland, F. D., Samet, J. M. (1994). Lung cancer. *Cancer Surv*, **19–20**, 175–95.

2. Lopez-Abente, G., Pollan, M., de la Iglesia, P. and Ruiz, M. (1995). Characterization of the lung cancer epidemic in the European Union (1970−1990). *Cancer Epidemiol Biomarkers Prev*, **4**, 813−20.

3. Boffetta, P., Trichopoulos, D. (2002). Cancer of the lung, larynx and pleura. In: *Textbook of Cancer Epidemiology*, Adami, H.O., Hunter, D., Trichopoulos, D., eds. Oxford: Oxford University Press, pp. 248−80.

4. Parkin, D.M., Whelan, S.L., Ferlay, J., Teppo, L., Thomas, D.B. (2002). *Cancer incidence in Five Continents*, Vol. VIII. IARC Scientific Publications No. 155. Lyon: IARC Press.

5. Feder, M., Siegfried, J.M., Balshem, A., Litwin, S., Keller, S.M., Liu, Z., Testa, J.R. (1998). Clinical relevance of chromosome abnormalities in non-small cell lung cancer. *Cancer Genet Cytogenet*, **102**, 25−31.

6. Girard, L., Zochbauer-Muller, S., Virmani, A.K., Gazdar, A.F., Minna, J.D. (2000). Genome-wide allelotyping of lung cancer identifies new regions of allelic loss, differences between small cell lung cancer and non-small lung cancer, and loci clustering. *Cancer Res*, **60**, 4894−906.

7. Mao, L. (2001). Molecular abnormalities in lung carcinogenesis and their potential clinical implications. *Lung Cancer*, **34**, Suppl 2, S27−S34.

8. Minna, J.D., Roth, J.A., Gazdar, A.F. (2002). Focus on lung cancer. *Cancer Cell*, **1**, 49−52.

9. Yokota, J., Kohno, T. (2004). Molecular footprints of human lung cancer progression. *Cancer Sci*, **95**, 17−204.

10. Toyooka, S., Maruyama, R., Toyooka, K.O., McLerran, D., Feng, Z., Fukuyama, Y., Virmani, A.K., Zochbauer-Muller, S., Tsukuda, K., Sugio, K., Shimizu, N., Shimizu, K., Lee, H., Chen, C.Y., Fong, K.M., Gilcrease, M., Roth, J.A., Minna, J.D., Gazdar, A.F. (2003). Smoke exposure, histologic type and geography-related differences in the methylation profiles of non-small cell lung cancer. *Int J Cancer*, **103**, 153−60.

11. Franklin, W.A., Veve, R., Hirsch, F.R., Helfrich, B.A., Bunn, P.A. Jr (2002). Epidermal growth factor receptor family in lung cancer and premalignancy. *Semin Oncol*, **29**, 3−14.

12. Hirsch, F.R., Franklin, W.A., Gazdar, A.F., Bunn, P.A. Jr (2001). Early detection of lung cancer: clinical perspectives of recent advances in biology and radiology. *Clin Cancer Res*, **7**, 5−22.

13. Wistuba, I.I., Gazdar, A.F. (2003). Characteristic genetic alterations in lung cancer. *Methods Mol Med*, **74**, 3−28.

14. Kawakami, S., Sone, S., Takashima, S., Li, F., Yang, Z.G., Maruyama, Y., Honda, T., Hasegawa, M., Wang, J.C. (2001). Atypical adenomatous hyperplasia of the lung: correlation between high-resolution CT findings and histopathologic features. *Eur Radiol*, **11**, 811−14.

15. Kushihashi, T., Munechika, H., Ri, K., Kubota, H., Ukisu, R., Satoh, S., Motoya, H., Kurashita, Y., Soejima, K., Kadokura, M. (1994). Bronchioloalveolar adenoma of the lung: CT-pathologic correlation. *Radiology*, **193**, 789−93.

16. Chapman, A.D., Kerr, K.M. (2000). The association between atypical adenomatous hyperplasia and primary lung cancer. *Br J Cancer*, **83**, 632−6.

17. Logan, P. M., Miller, R. R., Evans, K., Muller, N. L. (1996). Bronchogenic carcinoma and coexistent bronchioloalveolar adenomas. Assessment of radiologic detection and follow-up in 28 patients. *Chest*, **109**, 713–17.

18. Suzuki, K., Nagai, K., Yoshida, J., Yokose, T., Kodama, T., Takahashi, K., Nishimura, M., Kawasaki, H., Yokozaki, M., Nishiwaki, Y. (1997). The prognosis of resected lung carcinoma associated with atypical adenomatous hyperplasia: a comparison of the prognosis of well-differentiated adenocarcinoma associated with atypical adenomatous hyperplasia and intrapulmonary metastasis. *Cancer*, **79**, 1521–6.

19. Takigawa, N., Segawa, Y., Nakata, M., Saeki, H., Mandai, K., Kishino, D., Shimono, M., Ida, M., Eguchi, K. (1999). Clinical investigation of atypical adenomatous hyperplasia of the lung. *Lung Cancer*, **25**, 115–21.

20. Aguayo, S. M., Miller, Y. E., Waldron, J. A. Jr, Bogin, R. M., Sunday, M. E., Staton, G. W. Jr, Beam, W. R., King, T. E. Jr (1992). Brief report: idiopathic diffuse hyperplasia of pulmonary neuroendocrine cells and airways disease. *N Engl J Med*, **327**, 1285–8.

21. Travis, W. D., Colby, T. V., Corrin, B., Shimosato, Y., Brambilla, E. (1999). *WHO Histological classification of Tumours. Histological Typing of Lung and Pleural Tumours.* 3rd ed. Berlin: Springer-Verlag.

22. Roggli, V. L., Vollmer, R. T., Greenberg, S. D., McGavran, M. H., Spjut, H. J., Yesner, R. (1985). Lung cancer heterogeneity. A blinded and randomized study of 100 consecutive cases. *Human Pathol*, **16**, 569–79.

23. Travis, W. D., Brambilla, E., Muller-Hermelink, H. K., Harris, C. C. (2004). *WHO Classification of Tumours. Pathology and Genetics of Tumours of the Lung, Pleura, Thymus and Heart.* Lyon: IARC Press.

24. Tomashefski, J. F. Jr, Connors, A. F. Jr, Rosenthal, E. S., Hsiue, I. L. (1990). Peripheral vs central squamous cell carcinoma of the lung. A comparison of clinical features, histopathology, and survival. *Arch Pathol Lab Med*, **114**, 468–74.

25. Funai, K., Yokose, T., Ishii, G., Araki, K., Yoshida, J., Nishiwaki, Y., Ochiai, A. (2003). Clinocopathologic characteristics of peripheral squamous cell carcinoma of the lung. *Am J Surg Pathol*, **27**, 978–84.

26. Chieng, D. C., Cangiarella, J. F., Zakowski, M. F., Goswami, S., Cohen, J. M., Yee, H. T. (2001). Use of thyroid transcription factor 1, PE-10, and cytokeratins 7 and 20 in discriminating between primary lung carcinomas and metastatic lesions in fine needle aspiration specimens. *Cancer*, **93**, 330–6.

27. Chu, P. G., Weiss, L. M. (2002). Expression of cytokeratin 5/6 in epithelial neoplasms: an immunohistochemical study of 509 cases. *Mod Pathol*, **15**, 6–10.

28. Fukino, S., Hayashi, E., Fukata, T., Okada, M., Okada, K., Makihara, K., Morio, S. (1998). Primary clear cell carcinoma of the lung: report of an operative case. *Kyobu Geka*, **51**, 513–16.

29. Scarpatetti, M., Tsybrovskyy, O., Popper, H. H. (2002). Cytokeratin typing as an aid in the differential diagnosis of primary versus metastatic lung carcinomas, and comparison with normal lung. *Virchows Arch*, **440**, 70–6.

30. Cangemi, V., Volpino, P., D'Andrea, N., Puopolo, M., Fabrizi, S., Lonardo, M. T., Piat, G. (1995). Local and/or distant recurrences in T1-2/N0-1 non-small cell lung cancer. *Eur J Cardiothorac Surg*, **9**, 473–8.

31. Curran, W. J. Jr (2001). Therapy of limited stage small cell lung cancer. *Cancer Treat Res*, **105**, 229–52.

32. Nicholson, S. A., Beasley, M. B., Brambilla, E., Hasleton, P. S., Colby, T. V., Sheppard, M. N., Falk, R., Travis, W. D. (2002). Small cell lung carcinoma (SCLC): a clinicopathologic study of 100 cases with surgical specimens. *Am J Surg Pathol*, **26**, 1184–97.

33. Folpe, A. L., Gown, A. M., Lamps, L. W., Garcia, R., Dail, D. H., Zarbo, R. J., Schmidt, R. A. (1999). Thyroid transcription factor-1: immunohistochemical evaluation in pulmonary neuroendocrine tumours. *Mod Pathol*, **12**, 5–8.

34. Kaufmann, O., Dietel, M. (2000). Expression of thyroid transcription factor-1 in pulmonary and extrapulmonary small cell carcinomas and other neuroendocrine carcinomas of various primary sites. *Histopathology*, **36**, 415–20.

35. Shimosato, Y., Suzuki, A., Hashimoto, T., Nishiwaki, Y., Kodama, T., Yoneyama, T., Kameya, T. (1980). Prognostic implications of fibrotic focus (scar) in small peripheral lung cancers. *Am J Surg Pathol*, **4**, 365–73.

36. Koss, M., Travis, W. D., Moran, C., Hochholzer, L. (1992). Pseudomesotheliomatous adenocarcinoma: a reappraisal. *Semin Diagn Pathol*, **9**, 117–23.

37. Chung, C. K., Zaino, R., Stryker, J. A., O'Neill, M. Jr, DeMuth, W. E. Jr (1982). Carcinoma of the lung: evaluation of histological grade and factors influencing prognosis. *Ann Thorac Surg*, **33**, 599–604.

38. Miyoshi, T., Satoh, Y., Okumura, S., Nakagawa, K., Shirakusa, T., Tsuchiya, E., Ishikawa, Y. (2003). Early-stage lung adenocarcinomas with a micropapillary pattern, a distinct pathologic marker for a significantly poorer prognosis. *Am J Surg Pathol*, **27**, 101–9.

39. Noguchi, M., Morikawa, A., Kawasaki, M., Matsuno, Y., Yamada, T., Hirohashi, S., Kondo, H., Shimosato, Y. (1995). Small adenocarcinoma of the lung. Histologic characteristics and prognosis. *Cancer*, **75**, 2844–52.

40. Silver, S. A., Askin, F. B. (1997). True papillary carcinoma of the lung: a distinct clinicopathologic entity. *Am J Surg Pathol*, **21**, 43–51.

41. Lyda, M. H., Weiss, L. M. (2000). Immunoreactivity for epithelial and neuroendocrine antibodies are useful in the differential diagnosis of lung carcinomas. *Hum Pathol*, **31**, 980–7.

42. Sturm, N., Lantuejoul, S., Laverriere, M. H., Papotti, M., Brichon, P. Y., Brambilla, C., Brambilla, E. (2001). Thyroid transcription factor 1 and cytokeratins 1, 5, 10, 14 (34betaE12)

expression in basaloid and large cell neuroendocrine carcinomas of the lung. *Hum Pathol*, **32**, 918–25.

43. Pelosi, G., Pasini, F., Sonzogni, A., Maffini, F., Maisonneuve, P., Iannucci, A., Terzi, A., De Manzoni, G., Bresaoloa, E., Viale, G. (2003). Prognostic implications of neuroendocrine differentiation and hormone production in patients with Stage I non-small cell lung carcinoma. *Cancer*, **97**, 2487–97.

44. Gajra, A., Tatum, A. H., Newman, N., Gamble, G. P., Lichtenstein, S., Rooney, M. T., Graziano, S. L. (2002). The predictive value of neuroendocrine markers and p53 for response to chemotherapy and survival in patients with advanced non-small cell lung cancer. *Lung Cancer*, **36**, 159–65.

45. Schleusener, J. T., Tazelaar, H. D., Jung, S. H., Cha, S. S., Cera, P. J., Myers, J. L., Creagan, E. T., Goldberg, R. M., Marschke, R. F. Jr (1996). Neuroendocrine differentiation is an independent prognostic factor in chemotherapy-treated non-small cell lung carcinoma. *Cancer*, **77**, 1284–91.

46. Charles, J., Rossell, R., Ariza, A., Pellicer, I., Sanchez, J. J., Fernandez-Vasalo, G., Abad, A., Barnadas, A. (1993). Neuroendocrine differentiation as a prognostic factor in non-small cell lung cancer. *Lung Cancer*, **10**, 209–19.

47. Skov, B. G., Sorensen, J. B., Hirsch, F. R., Larsson, L. I., Hansen, H. H. (1991). Prognostic impact of histologic demonstration of chromogranin A and neuron specific enolase in pulmonary adenocarcinoma. *Ann Oncol*, **2**, 350–60.

48. Sudaresan, V., Reeve, J. G., Stenning, S., Stewart, S., Bleehen, N. M. (1991). Neuroendocrine differentiation and clinical behaviour in non-small cell lung tumours. *Br J Cancer*, **64**, 333–8.

49. Ishida, T., Kaneko, S., Yokoyama, H., Inoue, T., Sugio, K., Sugimachi, K. (1992). Adenosquamous carcinoma of the lung. Clinicopathologic and immunohistochemical features. *Am J Clin Pathol*, **97**, 678–85.

50. Guarino, M., Micheli, P., Pallotti, F., Giordano, F. (1999). Pathological relevance of epithelial and mesenchymal phenotype plasticity. *Pathol Res Pract*, **195**, 379–89.

51. Colby, T. V., Koss, M., Travis, W. D. (1995). Tumors of the lower respiratory tract. 3rd ed. Washington, DC: Armed Forces Institute of Pathology.

52. Beasley, M. B., Thunnissen, F. B., Brambilla, E., Hasleton, P., Steele, R., Hammar, S. P., Colby, T. V., Sheppard, M. N., Shimosato, Y., Koss, M. N., Falk, R., Travis, W. D. (2000). Pulmonary atypical carcinoid: Predictors of survival in 106 cases. *Hum Pathol*, **31**, 1250–65.

53. Fink, G., Krelbaum, T., Yellin, A., Bendayan, D., Saute, M., Glazer, M., Kramer, M. R. (2001). Pulmonary carcinoid: presentation, diagnosis, and outcome in 142 patients in Israel and review of 640 cases from the literature. *Chest*, **119**, 1647–51.

54. Thomas, C. F. Jr, Tazelaar, H. D., Jett, J. R. (2001). Typical and atypical pulmonary carcinoids: outcome in patients presenting with regional lymph node involvement. *Chest*, **119**, 1143–50.

3

Imaging of Lung Cancer

Sayed A. H. Z. Jafri and Sarah J. Copley

Department of Radiology, Hammersmith Hospital, London, UK

Introduction

According to estimates of the American Cancer Society over 170,000 new cases of bronchogenic carcinoma will have been diagnosed in the United States alone during 2005 [1]. Moreover, nearly 60% of those diagnosed with lung cancer will die within one year of diagnosis rising to a staggering 75% at two years and 90% at five years. Lung cancer remains the leading cause of cancer deaths worldwide in both sexes with an estimated 163,510 deaths (90,490 in men and 73,020 in women) predicted in 2005. It is a sobering thought that no improvement in survival from lung cancer has occurred in the last 10 years.

In the following chapter the imaging features of primary bronchogenic carcinoma, principally on chest radiography and computed tomography (CT) are considered; a separate chapter has been devoted to the utility of imaging tests in the staging of lung cancer in this volume. Although the histopathological features are also covered in detail elsewhere in this volume on lung cancer, the present chapter begins with a brief discussion of the pertinent histopathological considerations.

Histopathological Classification of Lung Cancer

The most widely accepted histological classification system is that of the World Health Organisation [2] which categorizes primary lung neoplasms into four common cell types:

Squamous Cell Carcinoma

This histological subtype accounts for 30% of all primary malignant lung tumours and it typically originates centrally. Cavitation with thick and irregular walls is a characteristic finding in up to 20%, particularly in those lesions which are peripherally sited and may be larger than 4 cm in diameter [3]. The incidence of this cellular subtype of bronchogenic carcinoma, which is strongly associated with cigarette smoking, appears to be declining, which may partly be explained by the increasingly strong anti-smoking drive in western countries [4].

Adenocarcinoma (Including Bronchoalveolar Cell Carcinoma)

Now arguably the most common histopathological subtype of primary lung tumour (accounting for 30–35%). The majority present as small (commonly less than 4 cm in diameter), smoothly marginated oval or round peripheral nodules. However, it is noteworthy that nearly one quarter of bronchoalveolar cell carcinomas may present as chronic air space [5] opacities typically with focal irregular opacities that may coalesce to produce consolidation within one lobe or even an entire lung.

Large Cell Carcinoma

Accounting for 15–20% of all tumours, large cell carcinomas are typically large, poorly defined peripheral masses with a tendency to produce early large volume hilar (30%) and mediastinal (10%) lymph node enlargement [6–8].

Small Cell Carcinoma

This subtype (which accounts for up to 25% of lung cancers) is thought to arise from neuroendocrine cells [9] and then to be central in up to 90% of cases [10]. There is a propensity for early mediastinal extension and encasement of vascular and tracheo-bronchial structures [11]. Compression of central airways secondary to mediastinal invasion or the characteristic early massive hilar and mediastinal lymph node enlargement, often gives rise to segmental or lobar collapse. Small cell carcinomas are among the most aggressive primary lung tumours with over 70% of patients having evidence of extrathoracic spread at diagnosis [12].

Rarer histopathological variants of lung cancer such as clear cell carcinoma, bronchial gland carcinoma and sarcoma are also recognized as are some mixed tumours (e.g. adenosquamous carcinomas). It is worth noting that the histological classification of primary lung tumours can pose problems due to cellular heterogeneity within an individual tumour and interpretive variation between pathologists.

Radiological Tests Used in the Diagnosis of Lung Cancer

In principal, plain chest radiography is often the first investigation to be requested in patients with suspected lung cancer. However, once a suspicious lesion is detected, more detailed morphological information is frequently required. Whilst magnetic resonance imaging has significant advantages (for example, no ionizing radiation and the capacity for multiplanar imaging) it is fair to state that CT remains the prime radiological investigation in evaluating suspicious intrapulmonary masses. At best, ultrasound serves a predominantly problem-serving role in the diagnosis of lung cancer.

Chest Radiography in Lung Cancer Diagnosis

Chest radiography (specifically the erect PA frontal radiograph, with supplemental lateral and lordotic views as indicated) remains the preferred initial imaging technique for patients with suspected lung cancer because of its lower radiation dose, widespread availability and relative low cost.

On plain chest radiographs, lung tumours tend to take the form of either central or peripheral masses, although 20% of bronchoalveolar carcinomas may present as areas of chronic air space disease [5]. Central tumours may cause hilar lymph node enlargement, mediastinal invasion or obstruction of one or more bronchi with distal segmental or lobar collapse. In some patients, presumably because of supervening infection, the appearances are more in keeping with infective consolidation [13]. Both atelectasis and consolidation changes may obscure the underlying tumour mass. However, it is the persistence of such findings that should alert the radiologist to the possibility of an underlying lung malignancy.

Mediastinal invasion by a central tumour results in a variety of radiological appearances, ranging from simple widening of the mediastinal contour to secondary changes with phrenic nerve invasion or superior vena caval obstruction. Peripheral tumours generally present as well-defined or spiculated nodules [14] although thick-walled cavities [15] occasionally with internal nodularity and air crescents may also be seen. It must be stressed that, in the absence of secondary signs such as rib destruction or chest wall invasion, there are no definitive radiographic features which accurately distinguish between benign and malignant masses. In this regard, the so-called superior sulcus or Pancoast tumour is worthy of special mention since there is typically either an apical mass or a more subtle area of asymmetric focal thickening which can easily be overlooked [16]. This lack of conspicuity is compounded by overlying rib and clavicular shadows and consequently these tumours are best evaluated on either computed tomography (CT) or magnetic resonance imaging (MRI).

The chest radiograph may also reveal a pleural effusion which either indicates pleural invasion, lymphatic obstruction or a non-malignant sympathetic response. Metastatic bone destruction is also a common finding on chest radiographs although the sensitivity of isotope bone scans in identifying osteolytic metastases is considerably higher.

A brief discussion of the issues surrounding plain chest radiography is pertinent. In general, a high kVp exposure, using an asymmetric film-screen combination has, until recently, been the preferred technique for routine chest radiography. At high kVp, the coefficients of absorption of bone and soft tissue are sufficiently similar and enable visualization of underlying lung through bone whilst preserving adequate penetration of mediastinal structures. The technique also requires a shorter exposure thus producing less movement artifact and sharper images. More recently, the advent of digital radiographic technology has seen a gradual replacement of conventional film radiography equipment in many departments of radiology [17]. Digital radiography has a number of advantages over conventional technology including the availability of reusable detectors, the need for lower doses, a more linear X-ray dose-response curve and the ability to post-process images.

Ultimately, the sensitivity of the chest radiograph in diagnosing lung cancer is dependent upon both technical factors and interobserver variation [23]. Suboptimal positioning, exposure and movement artefact can reduce the conspicuity of pulmonary masses but even in optimal conditions pulmonary masses smaller than 1 cm diameter are rarely seen [24, 25].

Computed Tomography in Lung Cancer Diagnosis

Computed tomography (CT) remains pivotal in the diagnosis of lung tumours. Its superior contrast resolution and the absence of anatomical superimposition enable precise localization of suspicious masses and superior lesion characterization. CT is able to delineate the morphological features of peripheral nodules such as a corona radiata (in which soft tissue spicules radiate into the surrounding parenchyma) and coarse spiculation, which are associated with a higher risk of malignant infiltration [26] (Fig. 3.1). Intratumoural calcification is also reliably demonstrated – most calcific foci represent calcified granulomas which have been engulfed by the tumour

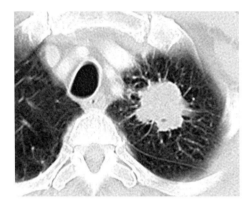

Figure 3.1 Non-small cell lung cancer. CT through the upper zone demonstrates a spiculated lesion in the left upper lobe

and are usually located in the peripheries of the mass [26]. Occasionally the calcification is more central in location with an amorphous character and represents dystrophic calcification within an area of necrotic tumour. Other features such as air bronchograms and ground-glass haloes [27, 28] and wall thickness of cavitating lesions (as well as the presence of air, fluid or tumour debris within cavities) are also well visualized on CT. The administration of iodinated contrast media may show differences in the avidity of contrast enhancement between benign and malignant lesions. Malignant lesions generally enhance to a greater degree than benign lesions (it has been suggested that an increase in density of $\geq$20 HU is 98% sensitive and 73% specific for a diagnosis of lung cancer [33]).

Enlarged mediastinal and hilar lymph nodes are well demonstrated on CT, as is chest wall invasion with soft tissue extension between ribs or rib destruction (Fig. 3.2). However, the utility and limitations of CT in the staging of lung cancer are more extensively addressed in a separate chapter.

With the advent of spiral CT technology a continuous (helical) volume of data could be acquired in a single-breath-hold scan. Single slice image acquisition was superseded in the late 1990s with the development of multi-detector row CT technology composed of multiple parallel detector arrays which simultaneously expose the region of interest thus acquiring a larger volume of data in a shorter time. The high quality multi-planar reconstructions available from these data sets have helped to establish the central role of CT in the staging of lung cancer particularly in assessment of resectability and mediastinal invasion. Furthermore, multi-detector row CT allows increasingly accurate measurement of the size of a nodule and assessment of interval changes enabling accurate estimates of tumour growth rates to be calculated using volumetric data [32]. In addition, post processing of volumetric data enables 3-D reconstructions to be rendered in real time,

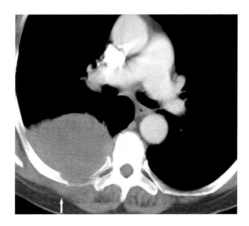

Figure 3.2 Peripheral right lower lobe squamous cell carcinoma. There is CT evidence of adjacent rib erosion indicating chest wall invasion (arrow)

for example, in virtual bronchoscopy where the data set is presented either using a surface shaded display or a virtual reconstruction technique.

Magnetic Resonance Imaging in Lung Cancer Diagnosis

Magnetic resonance imaging (MRI) has had a number of theorectical and real advantages over CT in the imaging of lung tumours not least the outstanding soft tissue contrast, inherent multi-planar imaging capability and absence of ionizing radiation. Unfortunately, these potential advantages have not been translated into real performance gains. A number of problems have proved difficult to surmount, particularly the low spatial resolution of the images and the inherently poor signal-to-noise ratio between tumours and lung parenchyma. Other issues include the suboptimal visualization of lobar vessels and fissures complicating the localization of nodules and motion artefacts degrading image quality on all but the shortest of sequences. In practice, despite the early expectations, MRI has not proved superior to CT in assessing the size of central tumours and is perhaps worse in identifying peripheral nodules. However, three areas in which MRI, was generally considered superior to CT (before the development of multi-detector row scanners) are worthy a mention:

(1) *Assessment of apical (superior sulcus or Pancoast) tumours.* MRI is potentially more sensitive in diagnosing chest wall invasion than CT [36] (94% versus 63% in one series [37]) and is better able to identify the presence and extent of bone marrow invasion, vascular encasement, brachial plexus involvement and extension into the spinal canal [38] [Fig. 3.3].

(2) *Chest wall invasion.* Unequivocal chest wall invasion is seen as well on CT as MRI and MRI is unable to resolve the pleural space. However, the extra-pleural

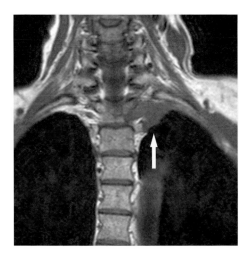

Figure 3.3 T1-weighted coronal MR image demonstrating tumour at the left apex (arrow) extending towards and into the T1/2 vertebral neural exit foramen

fat is clearly visualized on T1-weighted images with subtle infiltration more easily identified than with CT. Unfortunately the lack of signal change within extra pleural fat is not a definitive finding and, even if present, there is significant overlap between the appearances of direct tumour infiltration and inflammatory change caused by tumour abutting the pleura [39].

(3) *Pericardial invasion.* The pericardium is normally visualized as a low signal structure on ECG gated non-contrast MR and a breach is often relatively straightforward to identify [40].

Another area in which MRI may also have a very specific role is in assessing the degree of vascular invasion of mediastinal structures and in the investigation of complex pleural effusions in the context of pre-existing lung malignancy. Currently both CT and MRI have a low sensitivity and specificity for demonstrating mediastinal pleural infiltration and presently it appears unlikely that MRI offers any significant advantages over contrast enhanced multi-detector CT in the general assessment of mediastinal invasion.

Ultrasound

Because of the fundamental problem associated with imaging gas filled structures, ultrasound plays a minor role in the diagnosis of lung tumours. Occasionally, supraclavicular extension of Pancoast tumours or peripheral lung tumours which contact the pleural surface may be visualized and biopsied on an ultrasound scan, but the greatest utility remains in the aspiration of malignant pleural effusions to obtain cytological samples and relieve symptoms.

Central Versus Peripheral Tumours

The fundamental but practical division of bronchogenic carcinoma is between central and peripheral tumours. Up to 50% of bronchial tumours arise centrally (in or proximal to the segmental bronchi) with a further 40% originating more peripherally [41]. Characteristically, a central tumour produces obstruction of one or more central airways due to a combination of tumour encasement, mediastinal/hilar lymph node enlargement or direct endobronchial invasion. The appearance of a hilar mass with distal collapse, or less commonly, consolidation with superadded infection is the hallmark of a central obstructing tumour. By contrast, peripheral tumours often present as well defined masses with lobular or irregular spiculated margins. Rarely, the edges may be indistinct (giving the appearance of pneumonia) or mucous filled dilated bronchi (bronchocoeles) [42] may be identified. Most peripheral tumours also demonstrate air bronchograms or small round lucencies (pseudocavitatory changes) on CT however this is rarely evident on the plain chest radiographs [26]. Similarly a halo of ground-glass opacification may be found surrounding peripheral masses [27]. Both these features are more common with adenocarcinomas, particularly with bronchoalveolar cell carcinoma which may present solely as a focus of ground-glass opacity [43].

Peripheral Tumours

It is believed that around 40% of bronchial carcinomas arise from the bronchial mucosa beyond the segmental bronchi [41]. There are no reliable features that definitively distinguish benign from malignant peripheral masses. However, malignant masses are often larger in size and may demonstrate contour irregularities such as lobulation or spiculation.

Shape
Peripheral bronchial carcinomas are usually round or ovoid in appearance with well defined borders. Notable exceptions include superior sulcal tumours (a quarter of which present with asymmetrical focal pleural thickening) and tumours arising within scars or some bronchoalveolar cell carcinomas. Lobulation or umbilication is a common feature, [44] due to the differential rates of growth within the tumour. Less frequently, irregularity of the tumour edge may be seen due to the presence of multiple radial spiculations (corona radiata) which represents

either a desmoplastic response to the tumour by surrounding parenchyma or strands of tumour extending into the lung. It is interesting to note that when there is co-existent emphysema, a recent study has shown that presence or absence of spiculations cannot reliably distinguish between benign and malignant lesions [45].

Calcification

Calcification of lung tumours, whilst rarely appreciated on radiographs, is demonstrated in up to 10.6% of cases on CT [30]. The foci of calcification are usually eccentrically located and represent calcified granulomas which have been engulfed by the tumour. True dystrophic tumour calcification occurs in all cell types but is more frequent in tumours greater than five centimetres in diameter, although small peripheral tumours may contain ill defined amorphous foci [30].

Air Space Opacification

Focal cystic airspace lucencies are frequently found in all types of tumours but are most commonly seen in adenocarcinomas (particularly the bronchoalveolar cell variants). By contrast, air bronchograms are rarely encountered in other tumour types. A localized region of ground-glass opacification is often seen surrounding tumours of all cell types. However, again such a feature is most frequently seen on thin-section CT in adenocarcinomas, specifically the bronchoalveolar sub-type where 10% of tumours present solely as ground-glass shadowing [6]. It is an interesting fact that the proportion of an adenocarcinoma which is composed of ground-glass opacification has prognostic significance with increasingly extensive ground glass associated with a slower growth rate, lower levels of lymphovascular invasion and a better outcome [46].

Cavitation

Roughly 10−15% of peripheral tumours demonstrate cavitation on radiographs. As might be expected, the incidence of cavitation is higher on CT. Although cavitation may be found in tumours of any size or histological subtype, it is most commonly associated with squamous cell carcinomas and is rarely seen in small cell carcinomas. Characteristically, there is a thick (>8 mm) wall with an eccentric, often fluid-filled, cavity [15]. Rarer manifestations include nodules arising from the inner wall, an air meniscus or air fluid level, a smooth but gently lobulated wall or a thin wall of less than 4 mm (often due to extensive necrosis or tumour growth within a preexisting cavity) (Fig. 3.4). It is worth

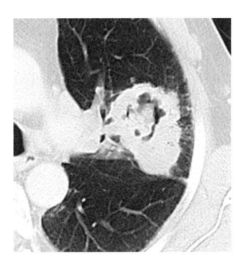

Figure 3.4 Non-small cell carcinoma in the left upper lobe. Targeted CT image shows a large lobulated mass with an eccentric cavity. The inner wall of the cavity is nodular and irregular

noting that a wall thickness of less than 1 mm indicates a benign lesion in 95% of patients, and a wall thickness of more than 15 mm indicates a malignant lesion in more than 80% of patients [47].

Growth Rate and Volumetric Analysis

Historically, a doubling time of between 1 and 18 months for malignant lesions has been derived from studies of radiographic follow-up in patients declining treatment of pulmonary malignancies; from this it has been extrapolated that a stable appearance over two years is strongly suggestive of a benign aetiology [48]. The evaluation of CT-based lung cancer screening programmes has led to the identification of a large numbers of sub-centimetre diameter nodules. The majority of these are unsuitable for biopsy, so the current accepted management is regular follow-up with a periodicity dictated by the size, shape, density and number of nodules detected [49]. There is a need to measure the growth rate of such lesions accurately. However, traditional 2-O orthogonal measurements are subject to significant errors and poor reproducibility with such small nodules (a doubling in the volume of a 5 mm nodule results in an increase of just 1.25 mm in its diameter [50]). This has led to the development of a technique called volumetric growth analysis; it utilizes computer-aided growth assessment based on thin-section CT scans with 1 mm collimation: nodule evaluation is improved by decreasing partial volume effects. Nodules of 5 mm or greater can then be serially reviewed and volume changes more accurately assessed than with traditional measurements of lesion diameter [50, 51]. The aim is non-invasively to distinguish between malignant and non-malignant pulmonary nodules at an early stage.

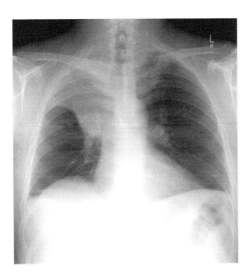

Figure 3.5 Golden's 'S' sign: there is dense homogeneous opacification in the right upper zone bounded inferiorly by the elevated horizontal fissure. Laterally the horizontal fissure is concave downwards. In contrast, centrally the fissure is draped around a large central tumour, and is convex downwards

Central Tumours

Central tumours classically present as a hilar mass and/or collapse or consolidation of the distal lung.

Hilar Enlargement

This is a common finding with up to 38% of patients presenting with a hilar or perihilar mass [52]. The hilar enlargement may be caused by the tumour itself or metastatic involvement of large hilar lymph nodes. Less frequently, it may be the result of focal lung consolidation or a mass superimposed over the hilum (often with a noticeable increase in the density of the hilum).

Collapse and Consolidation

Pulmonary atelectasis and consolidation may be due to a wide variety of causes but there are a number of suspicious radiological findings that are associated with an underlying central obstructing tumour [26] (Fig. 3.5). Specific features which should alert the radiologist to the possibility of an underlying neoplasm are listed in Table 3.1.

Bronchial obstruction leads to atelectasis and retention of secretions. However, the degree of distal opacification and volume loss may be less than expected due to collateral air drift or, more unusually, supervening infection. If obstruction persists, lipid-laden alveolar macrophages will eventually fill the alveoli of the obstructed bronchus resulting in an endogenous lipoid pneumonia (Golden pneumonia) and chronic inflammatory interstitial changes. On the radiograph the affected segments

Table 3.1. Features on chest radiography which may be considered suspicious of an underlying neoplasm

---

- *Persistent pneumonia*: a failure to improve over a period of three or more weeks in a patient at high risk (e.g. smoker or subject aged over 45 years)
- *Recurrent pneumonia*: repeated infection in the same lobe without evidence of complete intercurrent resolution
- *Golden's 'S' sign*: sigmoid configuration of horizontal fissure seen when the upper lobe collapses secondary to a central obstructing lesion
- *Significant hilar nodal enlargement*: relatively uncommon in the context of infection
- *Reduced airway calibre*
- *'Drowned lobe'*: Enlargement and opacification of a lobe secondary to the accumulation of secretions with or without supervening infection
- *Bronchocoeles*: mucous filled branching of dilated bronchi within a collapsed lobe

---

may demonstrate either a predominantly atelectatic or consolidative appearance but air bronchograms are best seen on CT.

The delineation of the central obstructing tumour may remain problematical in some cases even with CT or MRI (Fig. 3.6). However, in practice, the contrast enhancement characteristics of a tumour on CT are less than those of atelectatic lung [54]; T2-weighted or gadolinium-enhanced T1 weighted MRI images may show different signal characteristics between the tumour and collapsed/consolidated lung [55].

Cell Type-specific Imaging Patterns in Lung Cancer

Lung cancers may present with a multiplicity of appearances. However, the cell type often determines the radiographic pattern and may enables some inferences to be drawn regarding tumour histopathology. Small and large cell carcinomas have historically been associated with early hilar or mediastinal lymph node enlargement. Peripheral nodules are more likely to be adenocarcinomas, although large (>4 cm) tumour masses are more commonly associated with large cell squamous histology [6]. Peripheral squamous tumours retain their propensity for cavitation although without the consolidative or atelectatic changes typically found with central tumours.

Spiculation, ground-glass haloes, pleuro-parenchymal tails, air bronchograms and multiple cystic lucencies on CT are features most closely associated with

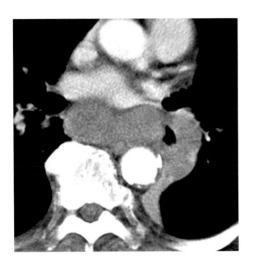

Figure 3.6 CT in a patient with small cell carcinoma. There is large volume subcarinal lymph node enlargement with circumferential involvement of the left lower bronchus and collapse of left lower lobe (note that only the apical segment is shown on this image), an appearance which may be regarded as a CT version of Golden's 'S' sign

adenocarcinomas but may be found in all cell types. However, pure ground-glass opacification without soft tissue density is characteristic of broncholoalveolar carcinoma (described briefly below).

Bronchoalveolar Cell Carcinoma

Bronchoalveolar cell carcinomas constitute between 2—5% of all lung cancers and are regarded as a subtype of adenocarcinoma with further subdivisions into non-mucinous, mucinous and mixed variants. They have unique epidemiological, pathological, and clinical features compared with other non-small cell lung cancers as, for example, there is no sex predilection and there is a poor correlation with tobacco consumption [56]. Consequently, there has been an increase in the relative incidence of the disease in recent years mirroring the fall in cigarette smoking [57]. Bronchoalveolar cell carcinomas often develop within areas of pulmonary fibrosis and scarring and most originate within alveoli or the most distal airways probably from either type II pneumocytes or bronchial epithelium. This largely peripheral origin helps to explain the common finding of areas of lepidic growth [58], which respect the normal anatomical boundaries and growth along the alveoli

There are two different radiological presentations of bronchoalveolar cell carcinomas. The most common is that of a focal solitary peripheral nodule which is often indistinguishable from other lung cancers. This appearance is more frequently seen with non-mucinous tumours. Thin-section CT may demonstrate a halo of ground-glass opacification surrounding the nodule but overt

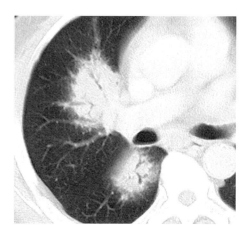

Figure 3.7 CT in bronchoalveolar cell carcinoma. There are two foci of dense consolidation (with haloes of ground-glass opacification) in the upper and apical segment of the right lower lobes

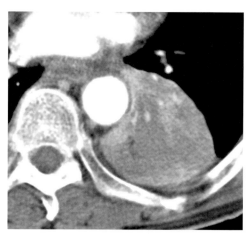

Figure 3.8 The CT angiogram: there are enhancing pulmonary vessels radiating into the collapsed left lower lobe

consolidation is usually absent. The prognosis of this type of tumour is significantly better than other lung cancers [59]. A less common manifestation of bronchoalveolar cell carcinomas is airspace opacification manifesting as either focal or diffuse areas of consolidation or multiple widespread ill defined nodules (more common with mucinous tumours). Air bronchograms are often a striking feature and the overall appearance may be indistinguishable from infective pneumonia. The prognosis with this pattern is, on average, poorer than the nodular variant [59] (Fig. 3.7). Differentiation between consolidative bronchoalveolar cell carcinoma and pneumonia, aspiration or pulmonary edema can be difficult. However the peripheral distribution, presence of multiple nodules and chronic history should suggest a malignant rather than benign aetiology. Other less specific signs suggestive of bronchoalveolar cell carcinoma include the presence of vessels coursing through the tumour on contrast-enhanced CT, the so-called CT angiogram sign [60] (Fig. 3.8). However, with fast helical scanners, this sign has also been seen in lymphoma and benign pathological processes such as pneumonia [61].

Conclusion

There have been a number of technological developments in the last few years that have impacted positively on the radiological diagnosis of lung cancer. The most significant of these perhaps has been the introduction of multi-detector row CT whose high quality data sets have led to the generation of fine increment volumetric reconstructions to assess tumour morphology and multiplanar reconstructions to delineate tumour extension into surrounding structures. The improved visualization of lung tumours has also led to more accurate volumetric analysis, which has in turn has allowed more accurate assessments of the nature of sub-centimetre pulmonary nodules to be made. Other advances have not been based on the refinement of pre-existing techniques but on sophisticated new methods of data analysis – the most significant example of this has been in the field of commercial computer-aided diagnostic programs to increase the sensitivity of already established imaging technologies.

Against the background of these paradigm shifts, other technologies that in the past were thought to hold great promise, have failed to find a wider role in the radiological diagnosis of lung malignancy: the role of MR is largely restricted to that of a problem-solving tool whereas US remains of dubious diagnostic utility.

REFERENCES

1. American Cancer Society (2005). *Cancer Facts & Figures - 2005*. Atlanta, GA: American Cancer Society.
2. Travis, W. D., Colby, T. V., Corrin, B., *et al.* (1999). World Health Organisation. Histological typing of lung and pleural tumours, 3rd ed. *International histological classification of tumours*, Vol I. Berlin: Springer Verlag.
3. Hansell, D. M., Armstrong, P., Lynch, D. A., McAdams, H. P. (2005). Neoplasms of the lungs, airways, and pleura. In: *Imaging of diseases of the chest* (4th edition). Hansell, D. M., Armstrong, P., Lynch, D. A., McAdams, H. P. (eds.). Philadelphia: Elsevier-Mosby.
4. Wynder, E. L., Muscat, J. E. (1995). The changing epidemiology of smoking and lung cancer histology. *Environ Health Perspect*, **103** (Suppl 8), 143–8.
5. Bonomo, L., Storto, M. L., Ciccotosto, C., Polverosi, R., Merlino, B., Bellelli, M., Guidotti, A. (1998). Bronchioloalveolar carcinoma of the lung. *Eur Radiol*, **8**, 996–1001.
6. Sider, L. (1990). Radiographic manifestations of primary bronchogenic carcinoma. *Radiol Clin North Am*, **28**, 583–97.
7. Theros, E. G. (1977). Varying manifestations of peripheral pulmonary neoplasms: a radiologic-pathologic correlative study. *AJR Am J Roentgenol*, **128**, 893–914.
8. Filderman, A. E., Shaw, C., Matthay, R. A. (1986). Lung cancer. Part I: Etiology, pathology, natural history, manifestations, and diagnostic techniques. *Invest Radiol*, **21**, 80–90.

9. Haque, A. K. (1991). Pathology of carcinoma of lung: an update on current concepts. *J Thorac Imaging*, **7**, 9–20.

10. Filderman, A. E., Shaw, C., Matthay, R. A. (1986). Lung cancer. Part I: Etiology, pathology, natural history, manifestations, and diagnostic techniques. *Invest Radiol*, **21**, 80–90.

11. Pearlberg, J. L., Sandler, M. A., Lewis, J. W. Jr, *et al.* (1988). Small-cell bronchogenic carcinoma: CT evaluation. *AJR Am J Roentgenol*, **150**, 265–8.

12. Micke, P., Faldum, A., Metz, T., Beeh, K. M., Bittinger, F., Hengstler, J. G., Buhl, R. (2002). Staging small cell lung cancer: Veterans Administration Lung Study Group versus International Association for the Study of Lung Cancer—what limits limited disease? *Lung Cancer*, Sept, **37**, 271–6.

13. Burke, M., Fraser, R. (1988). Obstructive pneumonitis: a pathologic and pathogenetic reappraisal. *Radiology*, **166**, 699–704.

14. Kuriyama, K., *et al.* (1987). CT-pathologic correlation in small peripheral lung cancers. *AJR Am J Roentgenol*, **149**, 1139–43.

15. Woodring, J. H., Fried, A. M., Chuang, V. P. (1980). Solitary cavities of the lung: diagnostic implications of cavity wall thickness. *AJR Am J Roentgenol*, **135**, 1269–71.

16. Johnson, D. H., Hainsworth, J. D., Greco, F. A. (1982). Pancoast's syndrome and small cell lung cancer. *Chest*, **82**, 602–6.

17. Schaefer-Prokop, C., Prokop, M. (2002). New imaging techniques in the treatment guidelines for lung cancer. *Eur Respir J Suppl*, **35**, 71s–83s.

18. van Heesewijk, H. P., van der Graaf, Y., de Valois, J. C., Vos, J. A., Feldberg, M. A. (1996). Chest imaging with a selenium detector versus conventional film radiography: a CT-controlled study. *Radiology*, **200**, 687–90.

19. van Heesewijk, H. P., Neitzel, U., van der Graaf, Y., de Valois, J. C., Feldberg, M. A. (1995). Digital chest imaging with a selenium detector: comparison with conventional radiography for visualization of specific anatomic regions of the chest. *AJR Am J Roentgenol*, **165**, 535–40.

20. Difazio, M. C., MacMahon, H., Xu, X. W., Tsai, P., Shiraishi, J., Armato, S. G. 3rd, Doi, K. (1997). Digital chest radiography: effect of temporal subtraction images on detection accuracy. *Radiology*, **202**, 447–52.

21. Kido, S., Ikezoe, J., Naito, H., Arisawa, J., Tamura, S., Kozuka, T., Ito, W., Shimura, K., Kato, H. (1995). Clinical evaluation of pulmonary nodules with single-exposure dual-energy subtraction chest radiography with an iterative noise-reduction algorithm. *Radiology*, **194**, 407–12.

22. MacMahon, H. (2000). Improvement in detection of pulmonary nodules: digital image processing and computer-aided diagnosis. *Radiographics*, **20**, 1169–77.

23. Herman, P. G., Gerson, D. E., Hessel, S. J., *et al.* (1975). Disagreements in chest roentgenogram interpretation. *Chest*, **68**, 278–82.

24. Kundel, H. L. (1981). Predictive value and threshold detectability of lung tumors. *Radiology*, **139**, 25–9.

25. Muhm, J. R., Miller, W. E., Fontana, R. S., Sanderson, D. R., Uhlenhopp, M. A. (1983). Lung cancer detected during a screening program using four-month chest radiographs. *Radiology*, **148**, 609–15.

26. Hansell, D. M. (2005). Neoplasms of the lungs airways and pleura. In: Hansell, D. M., Lynch, D. A., Page McAdams, H. eds. *Imaging of disease of the chest*, 4th ed. London: Elsevier Mosby (Harcourt), 785–899.

27. Kuriyama, K., Tateishi, R., Doi, O., Higashiyama, M., Kodama, K., Inoue, E., Narumi, Y., Fujita, M., Kuroda, C. (1991). Prevalence of air bronchograms in small peripheral carcinomas of the lung on thin-section CT: comparison with benign tumors. *AJR Am J Roentgenol*, **156**, 921–4.

28. Yabuuchi, H., Murayama, S., Sakai, S., Hashiguchi, N., Murakami, J., Muranaka, T., Soeda, H., Sugio, K., Nagashima, A., Masuda, K. (1999). Resected peripheral small cell carcinoma of the lung: computed tomographic-histologic correlation. *J Thorac Imaging*, **14**, 105–8.

29. Mahoney, M. C., Shipley, R. T., Corcoran, H. L., Dickson, B. A. (1990). CT demonstration of calcification in carcinoma of the lung. *AJR Am J Roentgenol*, **154**(2), 255–8.

30. Grewal, R. G., Austin, J. H. (1994). CT demonstration of calcification in carcinoma of the lung. *J Comput Assist Tomogr*, **18**, 867–71.

31. Ratto, G. B., Piacenza, G., Frola, C., Musante, F., Serrano, I., Giua, R., Salio, M., Jacovoni, P., Rovida, S. (1991). Chest wall involvement by lung cancer: computed tomographic detection and results of operation. *Ann Thorac Surg*, **51**, 182–8.

32. Yankelevitz, D. F., Reeves, A. P., Kostis, W. J., Zhao, B., Henschke, C. I. (2000). Small pulmonary nodules: volumetrically determined growth rates based on CT evaluation. *Radiology*, **217**, 251–6.

33. Swensen, S. J., Brown, L. R., Colby, T. V. (1996). Lung nodule enhancement at CT: prospective findings. *Radiology*, **201**, 447–55.

34. De Leyn, P., Schoonooghe, P., Deneffe, G., Van Raemdonck, D., Coosemans, W., Vansteenkiste, J., Lerut, T. (1996). Surgery for non-small cell lung cancer with unsuspected metastasis to ipsilateral mediastinal or subcarinal nodes (N2 disease). *Eur J Cardiothorac Surg*, **10**, 649–54.

35. Arita, T., Kuramitsu, T., Kawamura, M., Matsumoto, T., Matsunaga, N., Sugi, K., Esato, K. (1995). Bronchogenic carcinoma: incidence of metastases to normal sized lymph nodes. *Thorax*, **5012**, 1267–9.

36. Padovani, B., Mouroux, J., Seksik, L., Chanalet, S., Sedat, J., Rotomondo, C., Richelme, H., Serres, J. J. (1993). Chest wall invasion by bronchogenic carcinoma: evaluation with MR imaging. *Radiology*, **187**, 33–8.

37. Heelan, R. T., Demas, B. E., Caravelli, J. F., Martini, N., Bains, M. S., McCormack, P. M., Burt, M., Panicek, D. M., Mitzner, A. (1989). Superior sulcus tumors: *CT and MR imaging*. *Radiology*, **170**, 637–41.

38. Haramati, L. B., White, C. S. (2000). MR imaging of lung cancer. *Magn Reson Imaging Clin N Am*, **8**, 43–57.

39. Quint, L. E., Francis, I. R. (1999). Radiologic staging of lung cancer. *J Thorac Imaging*, **14**, 235–46.

40. Takahashi, K., Furuse, M., Hanaoka, H., Yamada, T., Mineta, M., Ono, H., Nagasawa, K., Aburano, T. (2000). Pulmonary vein and left atrial invasion by lung cancer: assessment by breath-hold gadolinium-enhanced three-dimensional MR angiography. *J Comput Assist Tomogr*, **24**, 557–61.

41. Auerbach, O., Garfinkel, L. (1991). The changing pattern of lung carcinoma. *Cancer*, **68**, 1973–7.

42. Aronberg, D. J., Sagel, S. S., Jost, R. G., Levitt, R. G. (1979). Oat cell carcinoma manifesting as a bronchocele. *AJR Am J Roentgenol*, **132**, 23–5.

43. Kuriyama, K., Seto, M., Kasugai, T., Higashiyama, M., Kido, S., Sawai, Y., Kodama, K., Kuroda, C. (1999). Ground-glass opacity on thin-section CT: value in differentiating subtypes of adenocarcinoma of the lung. *AJR Am J Roentgenol*, **173**, 465–9.

44. Theros, E. G. (1977). 1976 Caldwell Lecture: varying manifestation of peripheral pulmonary neoplasms: a radiologic-pathologic correlative study. *AJR Am J Roentgenol*, **128**, 893–914.

45. Matsuoka, S., Kurihara, Y., Yagihashi, K., Niimi, H., Nakajima, Y. (2005). Peripheral solitary pulmonary nodule: CT findings in patients with pulmonary emphysema. *Radiology*, **235**, 266–73.

46. Aoki, T., Tomoda, Y., Watanabe, H., Nakata, H., Kasai, T., Hashimoto, H., Kodate, M., Osaki, T., Yasumoto, K. (2001). Peripheral lung adenocarcinoma: correlation of thin-section CT findings with histologic prognostic factors and survival. *Radiology*, **220**, 803–9.

47. Woodring, J. H., Fried, A. M. (1983). Significance of wall thickness in solitary cavities of the lung: a follow-up study. *AJR Am J Roentgenol*, **140**, 473–74.

48. Yankelevitz, D. F., Henschke, C. I. (1997). Does 2-year stability imply that pulmonary nodules are benign? *AJR Am J Roentgenol*, **168**, 325–8.

49. Aberle, D. R., Gamsu, G., Henschke, C. I., Naidich, D. P., Swensen, S. J. (2001). A consensus statement of the Society of Thoracic Radiology: screening for lung cancer with helical computed tomography. *J Thorac Imaging*, **16**, 65–8.

50. Reeves, A. P., Yankelevitz, D. F., Kostis, W. J., Henschke, C. I. (2001). Volumetric growth index (VGI) for small pulmonary nodules: development and validation. Program and abstracts of the 87th Scientific Assembly of the Radiological Society of North America; November 25–30, 2001; Chicago, Illinois. *Radiology*, **221**(suppl), 311.

51. Ko, J. P., Rusinek, H., Naidich, D. P., *et al.* (2001). Wavelet compression of low-dose chest CT: effect on nodule detection. Program and abstracts of the 87th Scientific Assembly of the Radiological Society of North America; November 25–30, 2001; Chicago, Illinois. *Radiology*, **221**(suppl), 311.

52. Byrd, R. B., Miller, W. E., Carr, D. T., Payne, W. S., Woolner, L. B. (1968). The roentgenographic appearance of squamous cell carcinoma of the bronchus. *Mayo Clin Proc*, **43**, 327–32.

53. Reinig, J. W., Ross, P. (1984). Computed tomography appearance of Golden's "S" sign. *J Comput Tomogr*, **8**, 219–23.

54. Onitsuka, H., Tsukuda, M., Araki, A., Murakami, J., Torii, Y., Masuda, K. (1991). Differentiation of central lung tumor from postobstructive lobar collapse by rapid sequence computed tomography. *J Thorac Imaging*, **6**, 28−31.

55. Tobler, J., Levitt, R. G., Glazer, H. S., Moran, J., Crouch, E., Evens, R. G. (1987). Differentiation of proximal bronchogenic carcinoma from postobstructive lobar collapse by magnetic resonance imaging. Comparison with computed tomography. *Invest Radiol*, **22**, 538−43.

56. Greco, R. J., Steiner, R. M., Goldman, S., Cotler, H., Patchefsky, A., Cohn, H. E. (1986). Bronchoalveolar cell carcinoma of the lung. *Ann Thorac Surg*, **41**, 652−6.

57. Quinn, D., Gianlupi, A., Broste, S. (1996). The changing radiographic presentation of bronchogenic carcinoma with reference to cell types. *Chest*, **110**, 1474−9.

58. Cadranel, J. (2005). Bronchioloalveolar carcinoma. *Rev Mal Respir*, **28**, 570−5.

59. Okubo, K., Mark, E. J., Flieder, D., Wain, J. C., Wright, C. D., Moncure, A. C., Grillo, H. C., Mathisen, D. J. (1999). Bronchoalveolar carcinoma: clinical, radiologic, and pathologic factors and survival. *J Thorac Cardiovasc Surg*, **118**, 702−9.

60. Maldonado, R. L. (1999). The CT angiogram sign. *Radiology*, **210**, 323−4.

61. Sandomenico, F., Catalano, O., Cusati, B., Esposito, M., Siani, A. (1999). The angiogram sign in pulmonary atelectases studied by spiral computed tomography. Its incidence and semeiologic value. *Radiol Med (Torino)*, **98**, 477−81.

4

Screening for Lung Cancer

Thomas E. Hartman

Department of Radiology, Mayo Clinic, Rochester, MN, USA

Introduction

To screen or not to screen? That is the question! The current debate continues. Compelling reasons for both optimism and doubt about the effectiveness of screening have been voiced in the literature and at medical conferences worldwide. The aim of this chapter will be to provide some background on lung cancer, the rationale for screening and the outcome of previous screening trials. It will also attempt to frame the debate regarding CT screening for lung cancer by presenting its potential benefits and potential risks. It will then be up to the reader to decide his or her own position about CT.

Background

Lung cancer is the most common fatal malignancy in the United States and deaths from lung cancer exceed the combined total of breast, colorectal and prostate carcinomas which are the three next most common causes of cancer deaths [1]. It is estimated that 174,000 new cases and 160,000 deaths from lung cancer occurred in the United States in 2004. If mortality rates remain stable, over 1 million Americans will die of lung cancer in the next seven years. However, if there was an effective screening tool for lung cancer that resulted in a 10% mortality reduction an estimated 16,000 lives per year in the US could be saved. Breast, colorectal and prostate carcinomas all have relatively effective screening processes in place, which have demonstrated mortality reduction. It is these past successes for screening upon which the hope for lung cancer screening is founded.

Conditions for Screening

To screen effectively for a particular disease there are at least two conditions regarding the disease which must be met. First, there must be a phase during which the disease can be detected at a time when the individual is asymptomatic. The second condition is that there is an effective intervention during the presymptomatic phase that will alter the eventual outcome of the disease. In the case of lung cancer, the majority of stage I lung cancers are asymptomatic and it has been estimated that most of them have been present for at least four years before diagnosis [2]. Given these estimates it would appear that lung cancer meets the first criterion for screening.

With regard to the second criterion, previous survival studies following resection of stage I lung cancer have shown survival rates ranging from 62–82% [3–6]. Also previous studies of unresected stage I lung cancer have shown a survival rate of only 4% [2]. Therefore it would appear that lung cancer would also meet the second criterion in that intervention at an earlier stage may translate into decreased mortality. However, it should be remembered that survival and mortality are not equivalent terms and therefore the second condition has not been conclusively proved.

Prior Screening Trials

Before the advent of CT, the chest radiograph was investigated as a modality for lung cancer screening. During the 1970s there were three mass screening trials at Johns Hopkins, Memorial Sloan Kettering, and The Mayo Clinic [7–9]. In total over 30,000 men age 45 or older who were current smokers were enrolled in these studies. Not surprisingly there were more early stage cancers and increased 5-year survival in the screened cohort. However, these studies failed to demonstrate a mortality reduction from lung cancer in the screened group versus the control group. In this regard, it must be remembered that because of the inherent problems in screening studies (specifically, lead and length-time bias), there may be an increase in survival in the screened group but, importantly, disease-specific mortality may be unchanged. A Czechoslovakian study in the 1980s that involved over 6000 participants also failed to demonstrate a mortality reduction [10]. Finally, extended follow-up of the Mayo Clinic participants through 1996 showed no mortality difference between the screened and control groups [11].

Because of the inability to demonstrate an impact on mortality, the chest radiograph is not currently used for lung cancer screening.

CT Screening

Because the chest radiograph cannot effectively screen for lung cancer, investigators here turned to the use of low dose computed tomography as a potential screening tool. In a seminal study by Kaneko *et al.* [12], 3457 low dose spiral CT scans were performed on 1369 men, 50 years of age or older, who had a greater than 20-pack-year smoking history. The participants were imaged with both a chest radiograph and low dose chest CT. Chest CT detected a total of 15 lung cancers of which only four of the CT detected cancers were visible on the chest radiograph. CT was also able to detect smaller cancers with an average diameter of 16 mm whereas an average diameter for chest radiographs was only 30 mm. Another important finding from the CT screening perspective was that 93% of the CT detected cancers were stage I. This was much higher than the historical percentage of 20–25% potential resectable cancers.

Another important early study was the Early Lung Cancer Action Project (ELCAP) [13]. This study enrolled 1000 participants who were age 60 or older and had at least a 10-pack-year smoking history. Participants were imaged with both a chest radiograph and low dose spiral CT. A total of 27 lung cancers were detected on CT; however only seven of these were visible on the chest radiograph. Moreover, of the 27 CT detected cancers, 85% were stage I. These early studies showed the potential for CT to be an effective modality for lung cancer screening as it could identify more cancers and cancers at an earlier stage than was possible using the chest radiograph.

Mayo CT Screening Study

The results of a five-year prospective study utilizing low dose chest CT screening for lung cancer was recently published [14]. The Mayo study enrolled 1520 participants who were 50 years of age or older and had at least a 20-pack-year smoking history. Five annual CT screening studies were performed on the participants and a total of 3356 indeterminate nodules were identified in a total of 1118 (75%) of the participants. Of the total nodules, 2038 (61%) were less than 4 mm in size, 1034 (31%)

were between 4–7 mm in size, and 286 (8%) of the nodules were greater than 8 mm in size. There were a total of 1683 incidence nodules detected during the four years of incidence screening; 847 of them were not present on previous scans, while 836 incidence nodules were present. This meant that 25% (836/3356) of nodules were missed on the initial interpretation. A total of 68 primary lung cancers were detected in 66 of the participants. The 68 nodules that were found to be malignant were 2% of the total nodules detected and the 66 participants were 4.5% of the total number of participants. There were 31 prevalence cancers, 34 incidence cancers and three interval cancers. Twenty-nine of the 34 incidence cancers were non-small cell cancers and 17 (66%) were stage I tumours. Of the total nodules, the likelihood of a prevalence nodule being lung cancer was 1.2% (31/25.09) and the likelihood of an incidence nodule being a lung cancer was 4% (34/847).

It is these previous studies as well as others that have provided data which are both encouraging but, at the same time, have also raised questions regarding the utility of CT screening for lung cancer.

Reasons for Optimism

Previous studies have shown that CT can detect more cancers and smaller cancers than are visible on the chest radiograph and can detect them at an earlier stage [12, 13]. With effective intervention the hope is that the earlier detection will lead to decreased lung cancer mortality.

The improving ability to target appropriate populations for screening is another reason for optimism. Previous screening studies have identified a target population primarily based on age and pack years of smoking history. However, there are several studies currently underway looking at biomarkers in sputum, blood and urine in order to better target the population to be screened for lung cancer [15, 16]. A recent study has looked at exhaled breath condensate for the detection of lung cancer [17]. If this continues to show promise it could be incorporated into spiro-metry. With more effective targeting of the population to be screened, there is the potential to decrease the number of false positive exams. Given the large number of nodules detected at CT screening, it is important to be able to target the nodules most likely to yield a positive finding.

Studies by Henschke [18] and Midthun [19] have shown that for nodules of less than 5 mm, the likelihood of malignancy is less than 1% even in the high risk screening population. Additionally, even when these nodules were shown to be lung cancer at a later date because of growth, the vast majority of these were still stage I cancers. Therefore although the nodules would still need to be tracked, but a less aggressive follow-up of these smallest nodules would be possible.

For larger indeterminate nodules there are better tools available to evaluate these lesions short of resection. Nodule enhancement protocols on CT [20] and positron emission tomography (PET) [21] can be used to evaluate these nodules and have been shown to be cost-effective in decreasing the number of benign biopsies. Mass spectroscopy and other tools are under development which also show promise in decreasing the need for benign biopsies [22].

In addition to detecting lung cancers, other ancillary findings may be observed on screening images which can also result in mortality reduction. In the Mayo CT screening study 13 non-pulmonary malignancies were detected as well as 138 abdominal aortic aneurysms [23]. A consensus statement released in the *Journal of Vascular Surgery* in January 2004 judged screening for abdominal aortic aneurysm to be cost-effective [24]. These additional findings on CT screening for lung cancer may lead to additional overall mortality reductions.

There is also public demand for lung cancer screening. In a survey, public enthusiasm for lung cancer screening was not dampened by false positive test results or the possibility that testing could lead to unnecessary treatment [25]. In the setting of informed consent, if the public is aware of the limitations of the screening modality and still wished to proceed, should they be denied access?

Reasons for Doubt

Previous studies have shown that CT has the ability to detect more cancers and smaller cancers and to do so at an earlier stage than on the chest radiograph. The question remains whether this improvement relative to the chest radiograph will translate into improvement in lung cancer specific mortality. In a study of 61 CT detected lung cancers by Hasegawa *et al.* [26], it was found that 19 (31%) were well-differentiated adenocarcinomas. All 19 were stage I and the mean doubling time for these cancers was 1813 days or approximately 2.25 years. At this rate of doubling it would take a 3 mm cancer approximately 16 years to reach a size of 15 mm. Given that a 3 mm cancer is at the lower limits of CT detectability what is the likelihood that a smoker will survive 16 years as one of these well-differentiated adenocarcinomas grows to 15 mm? According to a national health interview survey [27], the average life expectancy of a 75 male past smoker is less than five years due to complications from smoking other than lung cancers, such as COPD, vascular diseases and esophageal carcinoma. With such a slow growing malignancy, the question arises whether these are cancers that the individual would die with instead of from.

In another study by Sone *et al.* [28] in a population of smokers and never smokers who were screened for lung cancer using mobile CT scanners, the incidence rate for cancer was 0.52% in smokers and 0.46% in non-smokers. This similar incidence rate raises the question whether the cancers detected in the never smokers are the same types of cancers that would lead to the same outcome as the cancer seen in smokers. In other words, could these be over diagnosis cancers.

If over diagnosis bias is present one could expect to see an increase in the number of stage I cancers detected, an increase in the resectability of the detected cancers, an increase in survival, and an increase in the total number of cancers detected. However, with over diagnosis bias there would be the same number of advanced cancers detected and there would be no decrease in overall lung cancer mortality. This set of findings was what was shown in the follow-up evaluation of the participants in the Mayo Lung Project that evaluated chest X-ray screening in the 1970s [11]. Therefore, it is likely that an over diagnosis bias existed in this study. Although the data for CT screening studies are still relatively limited, there are certainly findings that would suggest the possibility of an over diagnosis bias in these CT screening studies as well [14].

Although it has been shown that CT detected cancers are smaller and at an earlier stage, there remains a question of whether these cancers are being detected early enough for effective intervention. According to DeVita [29], the estimated average life expectancy of a lung cancer patient is approximately 10.5 years. At five years a typical lung cancer would measure approximately 0.4 mm in diameter which would still be below the ability of CT to detect. By 7.5 years the cancer would be approximately 4 mm in diameter at which CT would likely be able to detect it. At this point, however, the cancer would be roughly three-quarters of the way through its life expectancy and it may be that this is still too late in the course of the disease to alter the eventual outcome. Additionally, the majority of CT studies have shown that lung cancer detected by CT screening are closer to 10 mm in size and this would correspond to tumour age or approximately 8.5 years.

Additional questions regarding the potential timing of the intervention have been raised by studies that show that angiogenesis takes place in lung cancers 1−2 mm in size [30−33]. A study by Swartz [34] showed that per gram of lung cancer tissue there are approximately 3−6 million cells shed every 24 hours. A 5 mm diameter cancer has approximately a gram of tissue and therefore it is possible that CT may be identifying smaller lesions but lesions that are still too late in their life course for optimal intervention.

The large number of nodules which are detected at CT screening, most of which are false positives, is another potential problem. The workup of these nodules can place a significant burden on healthcare costs and can decrease the quality of life for the individuals who have an indeterminate nodule. Although studies have shown that the majority of these nodules are less than 5 mm in size, and therefore have a less than a 1% chance of being malignant [18, 19], there are still a significant number of larger nodules that would require further evaluation. Although CT nodule enhancement protocols [20] and PET [21] can be helpful in determining how aggressively to pursue some of these nodules, there is a false positive rate with both of these exams which may lead to more aggressive intervention than is warranted by the final diagnosis.

Surgical biopsy is still sometimes necessary for diagnosing determinate nodules and according to multicentre studies in Europe and the United States, the percentage of nodules resected which were ultimately shown to be benign has ranged from 46–52% [35, 36]. With the advent of CT screening more refined algorithms have been developed which have led to a lower benign diagnosis percentage at surgery (13–33%) [13, 14, 37]. However, this rate may still be too high for screening CT to be successful. A study by Romano *et al.* [38] that looked at the operative mortality rates in over 12,000 patients in community hospitals in California showed a mortality rate of 3.8% with wide resection. If one factors in the mortality from intervention in order to diagnose these pulmonary nodules it raises the hurdle for screening to overcome. For example, using the 2004 estimate of 174,000 new cancers and assuming a 25% benign surgery rate based on the CT screening studies, a total of 217,500 operations could be anticipated in order to resect these cancers. Using the 3.8% mortality rate reported in the Romano studies, a total of 8265 deaths from surgery could be expected. This is a significant portion of the 16,000 lives which would be projected to be saved by a 10% mortality reduction from lung cancer screening. This is simply an illustration and it could be argued that mortality rates of 3.8% are too high, however, it does illustrate the point that there is and will be associated morbidity and mortality with evaluation of nodules detected at lung cancer screening.

In addition to the mortality from surgical intervention there is also mortality associated with the radiation from the CT screening exam itself. In a study by Brenner [39] it was estimated that if 50% of all current and former smokers in the US who were between the ages of 50—75 years received annual CT screening, the estimated number of lung cancers caused by radiation from CT screening would be approximately 36,000. This would be a 1.8% increase over the expected number without screening. This study only took into account the radiation from the annual low dose CT screening exams, however; if additional low dose or conventional dose scans are performed between the screening exams to further evaluate indeterminate nodules, the radiation induced cancers would increase.

For all the advantages that CT screening provides over the chest radiograph there is still the question of cost-effectiveness and whether CT screening is an appropriate utilization of health care dollars. A study by Mahadevia [40] looked at the cost for quality adjusted life years. The study assumed that there was a 50% stage shift and a 13% decrease in lung cancer specific mortality. With these assumptions the cost to the health care system for quality adjusted life years saved would be $2.3 million for a former smoker, $558,000 for a quitting smoker, and $116,000 for a current smoker. Typically a cost of $50,000 or less for quality adjusted life year is considered the target for a cost-effective screening exam. While other studies using different assumptions have come up with different numbers, the question of cost-effectiveness will need to be answered because of the limited number of health care dollars available.

Conclusion

Lung cancer screening utilizing low dose CT shows great promise. Previous studies have shown that it can detect more lung cancers that are smaller and at an earlier stage. However, there are currently no studies which show a mortality decrease and this will be necessary before lung cancer screening with low dose CT can be judged to be effective. It is because of this a number of randomized control trials including the NCI sponsored National Lung Cancer Screening Trial [41] are currently underway. It is hoped that these studies can provide further clarification in regard to the effectiveness of CT screening in lung cancer. Some may argue that waiting for the results of a randomized control study may mean denying patients a screening tool that is ultimately shown to be able to save lives. However, others will argue that if money is spent screening with a tool that is ultimately shown to not be effective, we will have missed the opportunity to save lives had that money been directed to other areas of healthcare that are known to be effective.

REFERENCES

1. Greenlee, R. T., Hill-Harmon, M. B., Murray, T. (2001). Cancer Statistics 2001. *CA Cancer J Clin*, **51**, 15–36.
2. Flehinger, B. J., Melamed, M. R. (1994). Current status of screening for lung cancer. *Chest Surg Clinic N Am*, **4**, 1–15.
3. Pairolero, P. C., Williams, D. E., Bergstralh, E. J., *et al.* (1984). Postsurgical stage I bronchogenic carcinoma: morbid implications of recurrent disease. *Ann Thorac Surg*, **38**, 331–8.
4. Martini, N., Bains, M. S., Burt, M. E., *et al.* (1995). Incidence of local recurrence and second primary tumors in resected stage I lung cancer. *J Thorac Cardiovasc Surg*, **109**, 120–9.
5. Harpole, D. H., Herndon, J. E., Wolfe, W. G., Iglehart, J. D., Marks, J. R. (1995). A prognostic model of recurrence and death in stage I non-small cell lung cancer utilizing presentation, histopathy, and oncoprotein expression. *Cancer Res*, **55**, 51–6.
6. Gail, M. H., Eagan, R. T., Feld, R., *et al.* (1984). Prognostic factors in patients with resected stage I non-small cell lung cancer. A report from the Lung Cancer Study Group. *Cancer Res*, **54**, 1802–13.
7. Frost, J. K., Ball, W. C., Levin, M. L., Tockman, M. S., Baker, R. R., Carter, D., *et al.* (1984). Early lung cancer detection: results of the initial (prevalence) radiologic and cytologic screening in the Johns Hopkins study. *Am Rev Respir Disease*, **130**, 549–4.
8. Flehinger, B. J., Melamed, M. R., Zaman, M. B., Heelan, R. T., Perchick, W. B., Martini, N. (1984). Early lung cancer detection: results of the initial (prevalence) radiologic and cytologic screening in the Memorial Sloan-Kettering study. *Am Rev Respir Disease*, **130**, 555–60.
9. Fontana, R. S., Sanderson, D. R., Taylor, W. F., *et al.* (1984). Early lung cancer detection: results of the initial (prevalence) radiologic and cytologic screening in the Mayo Clinic study. *Am Rev Respir Disease*, **130**, 561–5.
10. Kubik, A., Parkin, D. M., Khlat, M., *et al.* (1990). Lack of benefit from semi-annual screening for lung cancer of the lung: followup report of randomized controlled trial on a population of high risk males in Czechoslovakia. *Int J Cancer*, **45**, 26–33.
11. Marcus, P. M., Bergstralh, E. J., Fagerstrom, R. M., Williams, D. E., Fontana, R. S., Taylor, W. F., *et al.* (2000). Lung cancer mortality in the Mayo Lung Project: impact of extended follow-up. *J Natl Cancer Inst*, **92**, 1309–16.
12. Kaneko, M., Eguchi, K., Ohmatsu, H., *et al.* (1996). Peripheral lung cancer: screening and detection with low-dose spiral CT versus radiography. *Radiology*, **201**, 798–802.
13. Henschke, C. I., McCauley, D. I., Yankelevitz, D. F., *et al.* (1999). Early lung cancer action project: overall design and findings from baseline screening. *Lancet*, **354**, 99–105.
14. Swensen, S., Jett, J. R., Hartman, T. E., Midthun, D. E., Mandrekar, S. J., Hillman, S. L., *et al.* (2005). CT screening for lung cancer: Five-year prospective experience. *Radiology*, **235**, 259–65.

15. Aloia, T., Bepler, G., Harpole Dea. (2001). Integration of peripheral blood biomarkers with computed tomography to differentiate benign from malignant pulmonary opacities. *Cancer Detect Prev*, **25**, 336–43.

16. Khan, N., Cromer, C. L., Campa, M., Patz, E. F. (2004). Clinical utility of serum amyloid A and macrophage migration inhibitory factor as serum biomarkers for the detection of nonsmall cell lung carcinoma. *Cancer*, **101**, 379–84.

17. Phillips, M., Cotarco, R. N., Cummin, A. R. C. (2003). Detection of lung cancer with volatile markers in breath. *Chest*, **123**, 2115–23.

18. Henschke, C. I., Yankelevitz, J. F., Naidich, J. P., *et al.* (2004). CT screening for lung cancer: suspiciousness of nodules according to size on baseline scans. *Radiology*, **231**, 164–8.

19. Midthun, D. E., Swensen, S. J., Jett, J. R., Hartman, T. E. (2003). Evaluation of nodules detected by screening for lung cancer with low-dose spiral CT. *Lung Cancer*, **41**, 40.

20. Swensen, S. J., Vigianno, R. W., Midthun, J. E., *et al.* (2000). Lung nodule enhancement at CT: multicenter study. *Radiology*, **214**, 73–80.

21. Gould, M. K., *et al.* (2001). Accuracy of positron emission tomography for diagnosis of pulmonary nodules and mass lesions. *JAMA*, **285**, 914–24.

22. Howard, B. A., Wang, M. Z., Campa, M. J., *et al.* (2003). Identification and validation of a potential lung cancer serum biomarker detected by matrix-assisted laser desorption/ionization-time of flight spectra analysis. *Proteomics*, **3**, 1720–4.

23. Swensen, S. J., Jett, J. R., Sloan, J. A., *et al.* (2002). Screening for lung cancer with low-dose spiral computed tomography. *Am J Respir Crit Care Med*, **165**, 508–13.

24. Kent, K. C., Zwolak, R. M., Jaff, M. R., *et al.* (2004). Screening for abdominal aortic aneurysm: a consensus statement. *Journal of Vascular Surgery*, **39**, 267–9.

25. Schwartz, L. M., Woloshim, S., Fowler, F-T., Jr, Welch, H. G. (2004). Enthusiasm for cancer screening in the United States. *JAMA*, **291**, 71.

26. Hasegawa, M., Sone, S., Takashima, S., *et al.* (2000). Growth rate of small lung cancers detected on mass CT screening. *Br J Radiology*, **73**, 1252–59.

27. Gentleman, J. F., Pleis, J. R. (2002). The National Health Interview Survey: An Overview. *EFF Clinic Pract*, **5**, 3.

28. Sone, S., Takashima, S., Li, F., *et al.* (1998). Mass screening for lung cancer with mobile spiral computed tomography scanner. *Lancet*, **351**, 1242–5.

29. DeVita, V. T., Jr, Young, R. C., Casellos, G. P. (1975). Combination versus single agent chemotherapy: a review of the basis for selection of drug treatment of cancer. *Cancer*, **35**, 98–110.

30. Folkman, J. (1995). Seminars in medicine of The Beth Israel Hospital, Boston. Clinical applications of research on angiogenesis. *N Engl J Med*, **333**, 1757–63.

31. Rak, J. W., St Croix, B. D., Herbel, R. S. (1995). Consequences of angiogenesis for tumor progression, metastasis and cancer therapy. *Anti-Cancer Drugs*, **6**, 3–18.

32. Liotta, L. A., Kleinerman, J., Saidel, G. M. (1974). Quantitative relationships of intravascular tumor cells, tumor vessels and pulmonary metastases following tumor implantation. *Cancer Research*, **34**, 997–1004.

33. Yang, M., Hasegawa, S., Jiang, P., *et al.* (1998). Widespread skeletal metastatic potential of human lung cancer revealed by green fluorescent protein expression. *Cancer Res*, **58**, 4217–21.

34. Swartz, M. A., Kristensen, C. A., Melder, R. J., *et al.* (1999). Cells shed from tumors show reduced clonogenicity, resistance to apoptosis and in vivo tumorigenicity. *Brit Cancer*, **81**, 756–9.

35. Mack, M. J., Hazelrigg, S. R., Landreneau, R. J., Acuff, T. E. (1993). Thoracoscopy for the diagnosis of the indeterminate solitary pulmonary nodule. *Ann Thorac Surg*, **56**, 825–30.

36. Kim, H., Lee, K. S., Primack, S. L., *et al.* (2002). Small pulmonary nodules on CT accompanying surgically resectable lung cancer: likelihood of malignancy. *J Thoracic Imaging*, **17**, 40–6.

37. Diederich, S., Wormanns, D., Semik, M., Thomas, M., Lenzen, H., Roos, N., *et al.* (2002). Screening for early lung cancer with low-dose spiral CT: prevalence in 817 asymptomatic smokers. *Radiology*, **222**, 773–81.

38. Romano, P. S., Mark, D. H. (1992). Patient and hospital characteristics related to in-hospital mortality after lung cancer resection. *Chest*, **101**, 1332–7.

39. Brenner, D. J. (2004). Radiation risks potentially associated with low-dose CT screening of adult smokers for lung cancer. *Radiology*, **231**, 440–5.

40. Mahadevia, P. J., Fleisher, L. A., Frick, K. D., *et al.* (2003). Lung cancer screening with helical computed tomography in older adult smokers: a decision and cost-effectiveness analysis. *JAMA*, **289**, 313–22.

41. Aberle, D. R., *et al.* (2004). National Lung Screening Trial (NLST). *A Research Study for Smokers and Ex-smokers*, NIH Protocol.

5

Staging of Lung Cancer

Zelena A. Aziz

Department of Radiology, St Bartholomew, and the Royal London Hospital, London, UK

Introduction

Thoracic imaging is pivotal in the evaluation of patients with lung cancer. As with most other cancers, treatment options and outcomes are dependent on stage and cell type. Uniform criteria for reporting the findings of clinical and/or pathological evaluation are important in the initial management of patients with non-small cell lung cancer (NSCLC) and consequently all patients with NSCLC are typically staged before therapy according to the recommendations of the International Staging System for Lung Cancer [1]. The treatment of choice for NSCLC, in the absence of disseminated disease is surgical resection. The primary aim of staging is thus to determine whether a tumour can be completely removed by surgery; clear surgical margins in resection specimens and the absence of tumour cells in resected lymph nodes being the prime determinants of local recurrence and survival [2]. The aim of this chapter is to review the role of imaging in staging lung cancer, focusing on CT (currently, the main imaging modality used in staging) and MRI. For the sake of completeness the technique of position emission tomography (PET) will be referred to but this imaging modality is covered comprehensively elsewhere in this volume.

International Staging System (TNM staging) for Lung Cancer

Before considering the role of imaging tests in staging, it is worth reminding the reader about the International Staging System for lung cancer. For the purposes of staging, lung cancer is divided into non-small cell and small cell types, reflecting the significant differences in natural history and response to therapy. The International Staging System for NSCLC stratifies disease extent in terms of prognosis [1], and is based on the TNM grading of the primary tumour (Table 5.1), regional nodes (Table 5.2) and distant metastases (Table 5.3) which was most recently revised

Table 5.1. Definition of primary tumour (T) characteristics in lung cancer according to the TNM system [1]

Descriptor	Definition
Tx	Tumour proved by the presence of malignant cells in bronchopulmonary secretions but not apparent radiologically or bronchoscopically
TO	No evidence of primary tumour
TIS	Carcinoma-in-situ
T1	Tumour of 3 cm or less in greatest dimension Surrounded by lung or visceral pleural No evidence of invasion proximal to a lobar bronchus at bronchoscopy
T2	Tumour more than 3 cm, OR a tumour of any size with: involvement of the main bronchus (distance to the carina is 2 cm or more), OR the presence of atelectasis or obstructive pneumonitis that extends to the hilar region but doesn't involve the entire lung OR involvement of the visceral pleural
T3	Tumour of any size with: direct extension of chest wall (including superior sulcus tumours), diaphragm, mediastinal pleura or parietal pericardium OR tumour in the main bronchus within 2 cm of the carina (but not involving the carina)
T4	Tumour of any size with invasion of the mediastinum, heart, great vessels, trachea, oesophagus, vertebral body or carina OR the presence of a malignant pleural/pericardial effusion OR the presence of satellite tumour nodule(s) within the ipsilateral primary-tumour lobe of the lung

Table 5.2. Definition of nodal staging in lung cancer by TNM classification

Descriptor	Definition
N0	No demonstrable metastases to regional lymph nodes
N1	Metastases to lymph nodes in the peribronchial or ipsilateral hilar region, or both, including direct extension
N2	Metastases to ipsilateral mediastinal lymph nodes and subcarinal lymph nodes
N3	Metastases to contralateral mediastinal lymph nodes, contralateral hilar lymph nodes, ipsilateral or contralateral scalene, or supraclavicular lymph nodes

Table 5.3. Definition of metastatic involvement by TNM classification

Descriptor	Definition
Mx	Metastases cannot be assessed
M0	Absence of distant metastases
M1	Presence of distant metastases (separate metastatic tumour nodule(s) in the ipsilateral non-primary tumour lobe(s) of the lung are also grouped as M1

in 1997. The eight stages have been devised to produce groups which reflect management options and survival (Table 5.4) [1, 3].

Stage I tumours are confined to the lung and visceral pleura, without nodal and distant spread (Fig. 5.1). When the tumour involves a main bronchus, the tumour is >2 cm beyond the tracheal carina. Stage I is divided into A and B depending on whether the tumour is T1 or T2. Stage IIA (T1 N1 M0) tumours are the same as IA but have metastases to ipsilateral peribronchial and/or hilar nodes or intrapulmonary nodes by direct extension of the primary tumour. Stage IIB tumours are either: (1) the same as Stage IB but with ipsilateral hilar nodal metastasis; or (2) T3 tumours which directly invade chest wall, diaphragm, mediastinal pleura or parietal pericardium without nodal or distant spread. Stage IIIA tumours encompass T3 tumours with ipsilateral hilar node involvement (N1) and T1-T3 tumours with ipsilateral mediastinal and/or subcarinal nodes. Stage IIIB tumours are T4 tumours, or any tumour that has spread to contralateral nodes. Stage IV disease is metastatic to distant sites.

In terms of the T, N and M descriptors, radiological imaging is usually directed at detecting irresectable disease (T4, N3 or M1). Differentiating T1 to 3 from T4 lung cancer and the detection of contralateral nodal and/or extrathoracic metastases is important as these typically preclude surgical resection or require additional chemo- or radiotherapy.

Small cell lung cancer is classified as limited (confined to one hemithorax but may involve contralateral mediastinal and supraclavicular nodes), or extensive, according to the requirements for radiotherapy fields [4]. Small cell lung cancer is generally regarded as a systemic disease and is usually disseminated from the outset. Thus, the major role of imaging is to determine extrathoracic spread. This chapter will only address the staging of NSCLC.

Table 5.4. Stage definitions, resectability and five year survival figures (%) for non small cell lung carcinoma [1]

TNM Subset	International system for staging lung cancer 1997	Resectability	Survival clinical staging	Survival pathologic staging
Carcinoma *in situ*	0			
T1 N0 M0	IA	Resectable	61	67
T2 N0 M0	IB	Resectable	38	57
T1 N1 M0	IIA	Resectable	34	55
T2 N1 M0	IIB	Resectable	22–34	38–55
T3 N0 M0	IIB	Resectable		
T3 N1 M0	IIIA	The treatment of Stage IIIA tumours ranges from surgical resection to nonsurgical modes of treatment and varies from center to center	9–13	23–25
T1 N2 M0	IIIA			
T2 N2 M0	IIIA			
T3 N2 M0	IIIA			
T4 N0 M0	IIIB	Stage IIIB tumours are not considered surgical candidates. In some centres, and in selected cases, pre-operative chemotherapy is given to 'downstage' the tumour	1–8	
T4 N1 M0	IIIB			
T4 N2 M0	IIIB			
T1 N3 M0	IIIB			
T2 N3 M0	IIIB			
T3 N3 M0	IIIB			
T4 N3 M0	IIIB			
Any T, any N, M1	IV	Irresectable	1	

Note:
Stage IIIA now includes mainly patients with N2 disease. This group remains extremely heterogeneous. There are differing prognoses for those patients with preoperatively diagnosed N2 disease (5-year survival of 9% for both pathological and clinically diagnosed disease) as compared with 'unforeseen' N2 disease (5-year survival of 24–34%).

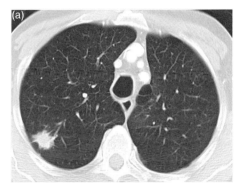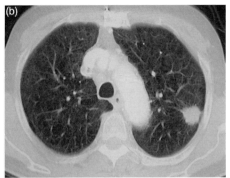

Figure 5.1 CT in two patients with T1 tumours. In both cases, the primary tumour is less than 3 cm in diameter and surrounded by lung. (a) 75-year-old male with primary adenocarcinoma of the right lung manifesting as a solitary irregular mass. (b) Tumour in the periphery of the left upper lobe with spiculated margins

Imaging Considerations

Chest radiography, computed tomography (CT), magnetic resonance imaging (MRI) and positron emission tomography using ^{18}fluorodeoxyglucose (^{18}FDG) are the imaging tests available for patients with lung cancer. Of these, chest radiography and CT of the chest remain the standard techniques used to define TNM staging. Chest radiography may permit a limited assessment of the size of the primary tumour and demonstration of features such as post-obstructive collapse and the presence of a pleural effusion. However, the chest radiograph is unreliable in detecting invasion of the chest wall, diaphragm and mediastinum and the presence of nodal involvement.

In contrast to plain chest radiography where there are issues of anatomical superimposition, the assessment of size and position of a tumour surrounded by aerated lung is generally more straightforward on CT. However, distinguishing between the tumour and collapsed or consolidated lung may occasionally also be difficult on CT (Fig. 5.2), leading to an over- or under-estimation of tumour size, chest wall or mediastinal contact. With contrast-enhanced CT, collapsed lung enhances more than central tumour [5] and may show mucus-filled bronchi, an indicator of collapsed lung. T2-weighted MRI can be useful for separately identifying tumour from distal collapse/consolidation [6, 7]. The tumour usually shows much lower T2 signal than the distal changes, and mucus-filled dilated bronchi can be specifically identified as high intensity tubular structures.

Table 5.5. Options for evaluating mediastinal lymph node involvement [84]

Noninvasive
   Chest radiograph
   Computed tomography
   Magnetic resonance imaging
   Positron emission tomography
Minimally invasive
   Bronchoscopy with transbronchial/transcarinal biopsy ($+/-$ endobronchial ultrasound)
   Endo-oesophageal ultrasound/fine-needle aspiration biopsy
Invasive staging
   Mediastinoscopy
   Mediastinotomy
   Extended cervical mediastinoscopy
   Video-assisted thoracoscopic biopsy
   Thoracotomy with intraoperative frozen section mediastinal sampling/dissection
   Mediastinal sentinel lymph node mapping

The detection of T4 disease is one of the main indications for the use of CT in staging lung carcinoma [8]. Despite better sensitivity relative to the chest radiograph, CT stage is discrepant with surgical findings in a substantial proportion of patients [9] with errors in overall stage occurring in up to 40% of cases [10]. Additionally, CT has not proved accurate in predicting the need for lobectomy versus pneumonectomy in centrally located tumours (which is based on whether or not the tumour has crossed fissures, invaded central vessels, or spread centrally within the bronchial tree). This decision remains a surgical one based on findings at rigid bronchoscopy or thoracotomy [9, 11]. Limitations aside, CT is a useful guide to surgical management and determines whether additional methods of preoperative staging are necessary.

Staging of Tumour Extent (T)

The T descriptor defines the size, location and extent of the primary tumour. Typically, radiological imaging is used to assess the presence and degree of pleural, chest wall and mediastinal invasion. Of particular importance is the distinction between T3 and T4 tumours as it reflects the dividing line between conventional surgical and non-surgical management. T4 tumours are considered largely irresectable by virtue of their involvement of vital mediastinal structures.

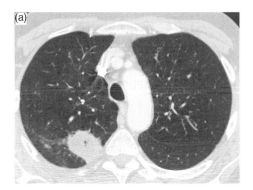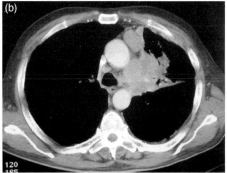

Figure 5.2 (a) Contrast-enhanced CT in a 70-year-old patient with proven squamous carcinoma of the right lung. The true extent of the tumour is difficult to define accurately due to the presence of surrounding consolidation. (b) CT through the upper zones demonstrating malignant mass in the aorto-pulmonary window. There is consolidation in the adjacent left upper lobe. However, the margins between tumour and consolidated lung are virtually impossible to define

However, surgical resection after induction therapy is occasionally being performed in a few selected patients with T4 tumour [12, 13]. Besides an improvement in locoregional control, patients who could be completely resected also showed an improvement in long-term survival rates that were unforeseen considering their initial clinical staging [12]. Primary tumours associated with 'satellite' nodules within the same lobe (as opposed to a nodule in a lobe other than the primary tumour which would be considered metastatic), are staged as T4 or irresectable disease (Fig. 5.3). However, it has been suggested that this designation may imply a worse prognosis than may be necessary. Consequently, some authorities advocate that patients with satellite nodules should undergo definitive resection if there are no other contraindications to surgery [14, 15].

Mediastinal Staging

Staging of the mediastinum either by invasive or non-invasive techniques should accurately determine whether patients are candidates for a potentially curative surgical resection, or for protocols involving multimodality approaches before, or instead of attempted surgical resection. Newer techniques to stage the mediastinum are rapidly evolving, and older techniques are being supplemented with information that stratifies patients into categories for the most appropriate therapy based on their prognosis. The most confounding aspect of the surgical staging of lung cancer involves accurate assessment of the mediastinum which should ideally define (A) mediastinal invasion and (B) mediastinal lymph node status.

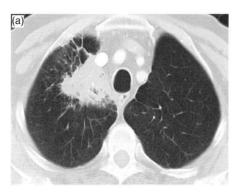

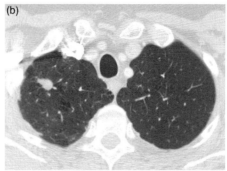

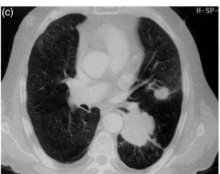

Figure 5.3 Male (54-years old) with primary T4 squamous cell carcinoma of the lung. CT demonstrates (a) an irregular cavitating mass in the right upper lobe associated with (b) a separate 'satellite' nodule in the same lobe. Both lesions were avidly positive on ^{18}FDG-PET scanning. (c) Another patient with squamous carcinoma of the left lower lobe with a metastatic nodule in the lingula

(A) Mediastinal Invasion

Both CT and MRI can demonstrate the presence of extensive tumour within the mediastinum. Clear-cut encasement of vital mediastinal structures such as the oesophagus, trachea, or major vessels, or deep penetration of tissue planes is conclusive evidence of a T4 tumour. Unfortunately, where lesser degrees of 'invasion' are present, criteria for irresectable (T4) disease are more difficult to define. Tumours that merely abut the mediastinum either alone, or in the presence of obliteration of, or interdigitation with, mediastinal fat planes, cannot be conclusively considered invasive (Fig. 5.4): loss of fat planes may reflect inflammatory change, fibrosis, or blurring from motion artefact rather than malignant invasion. CT features that suggest a tumour in contact with the mediastinum may be resectable include: (1) less than 3 cm contact with the mediastinum; (2) the presence of a fat plane between tumour and adjacent mediastinal structures; and (3) less than 90 degrees circumferential contact with the aorta [16]. Despite the use of these and similar criteria, the overall utility of CT for assessing mediastinal invasion has been disappointingly low.

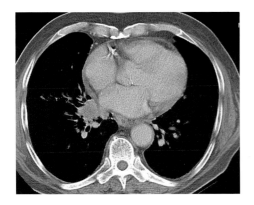

Figure 5.4 Male (80-years old) with a right hilar mass demonstrated on contrast-enhanced CT. The mass appears to abut the left atrium and there is associated pericardial thickening. PET scan did not reveal any nodal involvement or metastases. At surgery the tumour was completely resected

The advent of multidetector row CT (MDCT) into clinical practice has enabled better assessment of mediastinal invasion. Advantages include the ability to acquire thin sections in less time, more reliable contrast opacification of vascular structures, less artefact from cardiac and respiratory motion and limitation of partial volume averaging. Thin-section multiplanar reformats (MPRs) allow detailed assessment of important regions such as the carina, aortapulmonary window and the aortic arch. Early studies show that thin-section coronal reformats can improve the diagnostic accuracy of mediastinal invasion [17], although results of further studies are required before the advantages of MPRs in the crucial discrimination between T3 and T4 tumours are fully known. The use of MDCT acquired volumetric thin-section images (1.25 mm section thickness) has been shown to have a sensitivity, specificity, positive predictive value and negative predictive value of 86%, 93%, 60% and 98%, respectively [17].

Whilst the number of studies addressing the issue of accuracy of mediastinal invasion with MDCT is still limited and further data are awaited, it is recognized that the introduction of MDCT has allowed for a more confident interpretation of mediastinal invasion and may show definitively that the tumour is too extensive for resective surgery [18, 19]. MR imaging has the same limitations as CT with respect to differentiating tumour that simply abuts mediastinal structures from truly invasive disease. This is largely due to the inability of both techniques to reliably distinguish tumour invasion of mediastinal fat from adjacent inflammatory change [20, 21, 22]. Tumour invasion of the pericardium or heart may be better delineated on cardiac-gated MR imaging than on CT; the normal pericardium is of low signal intensity and disruption of the pericardium can therefore be recognized [23]. Direct invasion of the cardiac chambers is readily demonstrated on T1-weighted images because flowing blood in the cardiac chambers is depicted as

Table 5.6. Adverse prognostic factors associated with positive mediastinal nodes

(1) Extracapsular spread of tumour
(2) Multiple levels of involved lymph nodes
(3) Bulky, enlarged nodes
(4) Involvement of the higher, superior mediastinal nodes (nodes found positive at mediastinoscopy) compared to patients with a negative mediastinoscopy
(5) Involvement of subcarinal lymph nodes

signal void, and the tumour is conspicuous because of its higher signal intensity [24]. Cine MR images to demonstrate the presence or absence of a sliding motion between the primary tumour and adjacent structures may be useful to demonstrate invasion of the pericardium, cardiac chambers, main pulmonary artery and ascending aorta [25]. However, false-positive diagnoses may arise for cardiovascular structures that show minimal motion such as the distal aortic arch, descending thoracic aorta, SVC and pulmonary veins.

Overall, there is no objective evidence to suggest a significant difference in overall diagnostic accuracy between CT and MRI for distinguishing T3 and T4 tumours from less extensive disease and the routine use of MRI for the diagnosis of mediastinal invasion is not recommended.

(B) Mediastinal Lymph Nodes
The most important predictor of outcome in the majority of patients with NSCLC limited to the chest is the presence or absence of involved mediastinal lymph nodes. Adverse prognostic factors associated with positive mediastinal nodes are listed in Table 5.6. The position of lymph nodes should be described according to a standardized lymph node map. The preferred scheme is that adopted by the AJCC and UICC in 1997 (Table 5.7) [26]. Lymph node stations are defined by their relationship to fixed anatomical landmarks. Despite this, the distinction between lymph node stations, in particular, between hilar nodes (N1) and adjacent tracheo-bronchial (N2) nodes may be difficult. Mediastinal nodal metastases are often present at the time of initial diagnosis of NSCLC particularly with adenocarcinomas. Primary tumours > 3 cm (T2) and central, as opposed to peripheral tumours are more likely to be associated with nodal metastases.

Conventionally, patients with ipsilateral hilar (N1 disease) and mediastinal lymph node metastasis (N2) disease are considered to have potentially resectable

Table 5.7. Lymph node map definitions [1]

Nodal station	Anatomic landmarks
N2 nodes – all lie within the mediastinal pleural envelope	
(1) Highest mediastinal nodes	Nodes lying above a horizontal line at the upper rim of the brachiocephalic vein where it ascends to the left, crossing in front of the trachea at its midline
(2) Upper paratracheal nodes	Nodes lying above a horizontal line drawn tangential to the upper margin of the aortic arch and below the inferior boundary of No. 1 nodes
(3) Prevascular and retrotracheal nodes	Prevascular and retrotracheal nodes may be designated 3A and 3P; midline nodes are considered to be ipsilateral
(4) Lower paratracheal nodes	The lower paratracheal nodes on the right lie to the right of the midline of the trachea between a horizontal line drawn tangential to the upper margin of the aortic arch and a line extending across the right main bronchus at the upper margin of the upper lobe bronchus, and contained within the mediastinal pleural envelope; the lower para tracheal nodes on the left lie to the left of the midline of the trachea between a horizontal line drawn tangential to the upper margin of the aortic arch and a line extending across the left main bronchus at the level of the upper margin of the left upper lobe bronchus, medial to the ligamentum arteriosum and contained within the mediastinal pleural envelope
(5) Subaortic (aorto-pulmonary)	Subaortic nodes are lateral to the ligamentum arteriosum or aortal or left pulmonary artery and proximal to the first branch of the left pulmonary artery and lie within the mediastinal pleural envelope
(6) Paraaortic nodes (ascending aorta or phrenic)	Nodes lying anterior and lateral to the ascending aorta and the aortic arch or the innominate artery, beneath a line drawn tangential to the upper margin of the aortic arch
(7) Subcarinal nodes	Nodes lying caudal to the carina of the trachea, but not associated with the lower lobe bronchi or arteries within the lung

Table 5.7. (*cont.*)

Nodal station	Anatomic landmarks
(8) Paraoesophageal nodes (below carina)	Nodes lying adjacent to the wall of the oesophagus and to the right or left of the midline, excluding subcarinal nodes
(9) Pulmonary ligament nodes	Nodes lying within the pulmonary ligament, including those in the posterior wall and lower part of the inferior pulmonary vein
N1 nodes – All N1 nodes lie distal to the mediastinal pleural reflection and within the visceral pleural	
(10) Hilar nodes	The proximal lobar nodes, distal to the mediastinal pleural reflection and the nodes adjacent to the bronchus intermedius on the right
(11) Interlobar nodes	Nodes lying between the lobar bronchi
(12) Lobar nodes	Nodes adjacent to the distal lobar bronchi
(13) Segmental nodes	Nodes adjacent to the segmental bronchi
(14) Subsegmental nodes	Nodes around the subsegmental bronchi

disease. If contralateral mediastinal lymph node metastases (N3) are present, surgery is generally not indicated. The management of N2 disease is controversial. Certainly, surgery is considered to be inappropriate in symptomatic N2 disease, but the management of lesser degrees of N2 disease is more problematic. The heterogeneity of N2 prognostic categories may confound ongoing prospective trials attempting to define good-risk candidates for multimodality therapy. The heterogeneity phenomenon of mediastinal lymph node involvement was reviewed by Andre *et al* in 702 consecutive patients having surgical resection for N2 non-small cell lung cancer [27]. A multivariable analysis using Cox regression identified four negative prognostic factors: clinically apparent N2 disease, involvement of multiple lymph node stations, either pathological stage T3 or T4 status, or no preoperative chemotherapy. For patients having primary surgery, the 5-year survival varied according to N2 characteristics: one level node involvement with microscopic disease (34%) multiple level lymph nodes with microscopic disease (11%), single level clinically apparent disease (8%), and multilevel clinically apparent disease (3%). For patients with single level microscopic disease, there was no difference in survival between different lymph node stations [27]. This data reinforces the importance of knowing not only whether mediastinal lymph nodes are involved in NSCLC, but also the extent to which they may be involved.

With regards to CT, a size cut-off of 10-mm in short-axis diameter is most frequently used to distinguish benign from malignant lymph nodes. A recent review of 20 studies published since 1993 with a cohort of 3438 patients evaluated the accuracy of CT scanning for the mediastinal staging of lung cancer [28]. There was marked heterogeneity for the sensitivity (pooled value = 0.57) and specificity (pooled value = 0.82) with positive and negative predictive values of 0.56 and 0.83 respectively). These data reinforce the fact that findings on CT cannot be used solely to determine mediastinal lymph node status, and this remains the case despite improvements in CT technology. Obstructive pneumonitis with resulting enlarged lymph nodes can account for the fact that 40% of lymph nodes thought on CT to be malignant are actually benign, and microscopic involvement of lymph nodes is encountered in up to 15% of patients who undergo complete mediastinal lymph node dissection for presumed stage I disease [28]. One method of reducing the frequency of false-positive interpretations is to ensure that nodes draining the tumour are larger than nodes elsewhere in the mediastinum. By only counting enlarged nodes (>10 mm short axis diameter) that were at least 5 mm greater in diameter than nodes in regions not draining the tumour, Buy et al. were able to achieve a 95% positive predictive value for nodal metastatic disease [29].

The use of MRI for staging nodal disease relies, like CT on recognizing nodal enlargement. The considerable overlap of the T1 and T2 relaxation times of benign and malignant lymph nodes prevents the use of unenhanced MR signal intensity for tissue characterization [20, 30]. Intravenous contrast has not proved useful in distinguishing chronic inflammation from neoplastic involvement. The introduction of new lymph node specific contrast agents is a promising development. Ultrasmall superparamagnetic ironoxide nanparticles (USPIO) traverse the vascular endothelium and are phagocytosed by macrophages in normally functioning lymph nodes. This results in uniform signal loss in T2 and $T2^*$ weighted images and allows the differentiation of enlarged hyperplastic nodes from enlarged neoplastic nodes [31]. Based on early studies, a problem appears to be that not all inflammatory nodes show signal loss, and there are also false negative results [32]. Formal evaluation of sensitivity and specificity of this technique is awaited.

More recently, minimally invasive techniques such as bronchoscopy with transbronchial biopsy +/− endobronchial ultrasound and endo-oesophageal ultrasound with fine-needle aspiration (EUS-FNA) have been used to evaluate mediastinal lymph nodes. Endoscopic ultrasonography of the oesophagus allows excellent visualization of the mediastinum, particularly of the left-sided mediastinal lymph nodes and the subcarinal space. The procedure takes anatomical advantage of the fact that the oesophagus lies posteriorly and to the left of the trachea and is in the proximity of the lymph nodes between these two structures. Lymph node level 5 (aortopulmonary window), level 7 (subcarinal) and inferior mediastinal lymph nodes are particularly easy to access by this method, however, the views of the paratracheal and anterior mediastinal areas are limited by distortion caused by tracheal air. Wiersema *et al.* [33] recently reported the EUS-FNA was superior to transbronchial needle aspiration (TBNA) in the diagnosis of mediastinal metastases in NSCLC. Fritscher-Ravens *et al.* compared CT, PET and aspiration (EUS-FNA) for detection of mediastinal metastases in potentially resectable patients with lung cancer [34]. Their study concluded that EUS-FNA is more accurate than both CT and PET in detecting abnormal lymph nodes in the mediastinum. However, it must be emphasized that the role of hybrid PET/Ct images was not evaluated in this study. When performed in patients with enlarged lymph nodes, EUS-FNA has a reported sensitivity and specificity of between 85–93% and 91–100%, respectively [28, 35, 36]. EUS-FNA can also detect malignancy in normal-sized lymph nodes, and when successful has altered the staging in 18–42% of such patients [37, 38]. However the sensitivity and specificity are low with normal-sized lymph nodes due to the necessity of performing several aspirations from different sites in order to increase yield [38].

PET and PET/CT are increasingly being used for the staging of nodal metastases; the role of PET is discussed in detail in a separate chapter in this volume.

In summary, CT is still the first imaging modality used in assessing mediastinal lymph node status. In patients who are otherwise surgical candidates and where PET is available, PET is recommended as the next investigation [39]. If both the CT and PET findings are negative for mediastinal lymph node involvement, an argument can be made to proceed directly to surgery. However, if the CT and/or PET suggest nodal involvement, then some would favour TBNA or EUS-FNA for confirmation of malignant spread to the mediastinum. However, in these situations, mediastinoscopy is still performed to ascertain spread as the techniques of TBNA and EUS-FNA are still not utilized widely. It must be remembered that negative PET scanning does not preclude biopsy of radiographically-enlarged mediastinal lymph nodes and invasive sampling is necessary when the results of CT and FDG = PET do not corroborate each other.

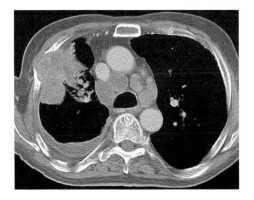

Figure 5.5 Male (64-years old) with a large necrotic mass (squamous cell carcinoma) within the right upper lobe. There is clear CT evidence of chest wall invasion with bone destruction and extension of tumour beyond the ribs. Extensive mediastinal lymphadenopathy and a pleural effusion are also seen

Chest Wall Invasion

A peripheral lung tumour may cross the parietal pleura and invade ribs and intercostal muscles. Such localized invasion of the chest wall (T3) by NSCLC does not necessarily preclude surgery, however, the mortality rate associated with en bloc resection of the tumour and contiguous structures remains substantial, so information about chest wall invasion is still an important factor in the clinical decision to perform surgery. With CT, the only findings with a high positive predictive value are rib destruction adjacent to a tumour mass or extension of tumour beyond ribs into the chest wall (Figs 5.5 and 5.6) [40]. Contact with the chest wall parietal pleura does not imply invasion even when associated with pleural thickening, although the more extensive the abnormality, the more likely it is that invasion has occurred [41]. As with the mediastinal pleura, parietal pleural thickening is a non-specific finding that may be secondary to reactive fibrosis or inflammation. The angle of contact between tumour and chest wall, obliteration of the extrapleural fat plane and the presence of extrapleural soft tissue are also unreliable signs of invasion [41−45]. Preservation of the extrapleural fat line is reassuring, but does not invariably exclude invasive disease [42]. MR does not confer any advantages for the assessment of chest wall invasion again because of the overlap in appearances between tumour extension and associated inflammatory change.

Both CT and MR have been used to apply dynamic imaging to assess the respiratory shift, defined as a change in the relative location between the peripheral lung tumour and the chest wall, during the respiratory cycle [46, 47]. A significant limitation of this technique (applicable to both CT and MR) is the fact that only absence of tumour invasion can be diagnosed; free movement of the tumour proves lack of attachment between the parietal and visceral pleura. Benign fibrous

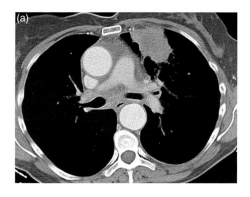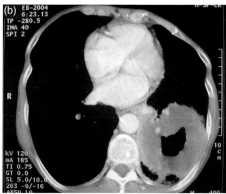

Figure 5.6 Two patients with non-small cell lung cancer. (a) Contrast enhanced CT demonstrates a peripheral mass within the lingula which abuts the left anterior chest wall. There are no definitive signs of chest wall invasion on CT (a conclusion confirmed at surgery). (b) Squamous carcinoma in the left lower lobe which appears intimately related to the postero-lateral chest wall. However, at surgery, there was no evidence of chest wall invasion at this site

adhesions may cause false-positive results by simulating tumour infiltration. In practical terms, these techniques are not widely available or practised, and currently, unless definite chest wall invasion is demonstrated on CT most patients will be referred for consideration of surgery if there are no other precluding factors.

Superior Sulcus Tumours

Superior sulcus tumours may be of any cell type [48, 49] and have a tendency to invade the adjacent chest wall and spine and to extend superiorly to involve the subclavian vessels and brachial plexus. Such tumours may be technically resectable, and accurate assessment of the local extent of disease is an important part of staging [50]. On chest radiography, in the absence of serial radiographs, distinguishing a superior sulcus tumour from apical pleural thickening may be difficult, unless there is obvious bone destruction, a feature that is seen on chest radiographs in approximately one-third of cases [51] (Fig. 5.7). MRI is currently regarded as the optimal modality for demonstrating the extent of superior sulcus tumours largely to demonstrate invasion of the brachial plexus, subclavian vessels, neural foramina and bone marrow [52–55]. In addition, disruption of the extrapleural fat line on MRI is a good indicator of chest wall invasion. High-quality volumetric MDCT with thin sections, bolus injection of contrast and sagittal and coronal reformats may provide the same information regarding the relationship of tumour to the

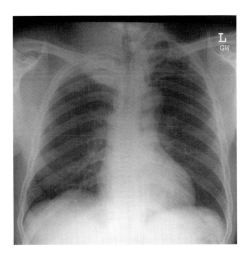

Figure 5.7 Patient (78-year-old) presenting with right arm pain and a Pancoast (superior sulcus) tumour at the right apex. There is a soft-tissue density opacity and clear evidence of first rib destruction

brachial plexus but studies comparing MDCT and MRI in the evaluation of superior sulcus tumours are at present lacking.

Extrathoracic Metastatic Disease

Distant metastases (M1) occur in 11 to 36% of patients with NSCLC with common sites being the adrenal glands, liver, brain, bones and abdominal lymph nodes. Although the approach to the detection of occult metastases remains controversial, a reasonable strategy for patients with no clinical features to suggest extrathoracic metastases is to extend the staging chest CT to include the liver and adrenal glands [56]. In most centres, no other routine imaging is undertaken. As distant metastases have been reported to be as low as 0—17% with a T1 primary malignancy in the absence of nodal metastases [40, 57], it has even been suggested that in patients with T1 to 2, N0 disease, imaging for occult extrathoracic metastases is not warranted [57, 58]. Whole body FDG-PET is increasingly being used to improve the accuracy of staging as it has been shown to have a higher sensitivity and specificity than CT, MRI and other radionuclide procedures for all body sites, apart from the brain in detecting metastases to the adrenals, bones and extrathoracic lymph nodes [59]. The use of whole body PET is likely to change the approach to diagnosing asymptomatic extrathoracic metastases.

Adrenal Metastases

The majority of unilateral adrenal masses in patients with lung cancer are benign but are difficult to distinguish from adrenal metastases. Adrenal metastases are

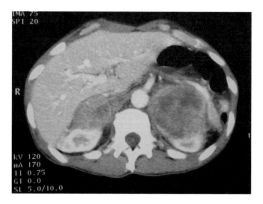

Figure 5.8 Adrenal metastases in a patient with proven non-small cell carcinoma of the lung. There are huge bilateral adrenal masses seen on the staging CT study

detected in up to 20% of patients with NSCLC at presentation [60–62] (Fig. 5.8). Findings from several studies have confirmed the usefulness of CT attenuation measurements at both unenhanced and delayed contrast-enhanced CT to differentiate benign from malignant lesions. Unlike metastases, adrenal adenomas often contain intracytoplasmic lipid in the adrenal cortex and thus demonstrate low attenuation at unenhanced CT. Boland *et al.* performed a meta-analysis of 10 CT studies and concluded that a threshold of 10 HU or less on unenhanced CT corresponded to a sensitivity of 71% and a specificity of 98% in the diagnosis of adrenal adenomas [63]. However, 29% of adenomas have attenuation values higher than 10HU (hyperattenuating) and remain indeterminate [64]. Delayed contrast-enhanced CT attenuation (10–15 minutes after contrast material injection) has been used successfully to differentiate adenomas from metastases. Adenomas demonstrate rapid washout after administration of intravenous contrast medium. At 10 minutes after injection of contrast, an attenuation value of less than 30 HU is diagnostic of an adenoma [65]. Additionally, a relative percentage washout higher than 40% or 50% at delayed contrast-enhanced CT has been found to be accurate in the diagnosis of adrenal adenomas. In clinical practice, the majority of adrenal masses are detected incidentally at contrast-enhanced CT. Unenhanced CT scans are not obtained routinely and patients frequently leave the radiology department before the contrast-enhanced examinations are reviewed. Mean CT-attenuation of adrenal masses at contrast-enhanced CT has limited usefulness because there is too much overlap between the two groups to allow accurate differentiation between adrenal adenomas and non-adenomas.

If the primary tumour is deemed operable by CT staging, then FDG-PET is useful in equivocal adrenal lesions identified on CT. Consequently, if FDG uptake by an adrenal mass is normal in a patient with potentially resectable disease, curative resection should be considered without further evaluation. Patients with NSCLC and an isolated adrenal mass with increased FDG uptake should have the lesion biopsied before being denied surgery.

An alternative option is to perform in-phase, out-of-phase MRI imaging to clarify lesions picked up during the initial staging CT. On MRI imaging, visual assessment of adrenal nodules using chemical shift imaging may characterize a nodule as an adenoma on the basis of a decrease in signal intensity of the nodule on out-of-phase imaging as compared with in phase imaging. Korobkin *et al.* applied this technique to 51 adrenal lesions and reported a sensitivity of 100% and specificity of 81% in characterizing adenomas [66]. In certain circumstances, chemical shift MR imaging is a reasonable second imaging test for further characterization of a hyperattenuating adrenal mass.

Image guided percutaneous aspiration biopsy may be performed for definitive diagnosis.

Hepatic Metastases

Most liver lesions encountered in patients with NSCLC are benign cysts or haemangiomas, with metastases being detected in 2.3% to 16% of patients at time of diagnosis [40, 67]. A meta-analysis that evaluated the utility of imaging in asymptomatic patients with NSCLC showed a pooled yield of only 3% in detecting hepatic metastases [68]. Although there has been marked qualitative improvement in imaging since this meta-analysis, it is a fact that hepatic metastases typically occur when there is locally advanced, inoperable intrathoracic disease and/or metastases to other organs [40]. In those rare patients who are potential candidates for curative resection with a hepatic lesion detected on CT of the chest that is indeterminate in aetiology, MR imaging or biopsy can be performed. Various MR imaging techniques have been used to distinguish benign lesions from metastases. The advent of liver-specific contrast agents targeted at hepatocytes or Kupffer cells has facilitated MR detection of hepatic metastases [69].

Brain Metastases

Metastases to the brain are more frequent when the primary tumour is greater than 3 cm [70] and more frequent for adenocarcinomas than for squamous cell carcinoma [58]. Routine brain imaging in the absence of symptoms or clinical signs is not recommended as the pick-up of occult cerebral metastases is reported to be between 2–4% [68], with a false-positive rate in one study of 11% [71].

Colice and co-workers performed a cost analysis and concluded that head CT should be reserved for those patients with abnormal neurological symptoms and signs [72]. However this conclusion has been challenged as it is based on data that may be skewed by a high proportion of patients with early stage disease who are at low risk for brain metastases. It has been shown that there is a substantial early postoperative recurrence in patients with non-squamous cell histology and stage of disease higher than T1 N0, suggesting that undetected metastases were present at the time of surgical resection of the primary lung malignancy [73−75]. Additionally Earnest and co-workers have reported that occult brain metastases were identified in 6 of 27 (22%) patients with potentially resectable NSCLC (excluding early stage lung cancer) on contrast-enhanced MR images [70]. Consequently, although the 1997 joint ATS/ERS statement on pre-treatment evaluation of NSCLC does not advocate the preoperative imaging of the brain in asymptomatic patients with NSCLC [76], there may be a limited role for imaging in the detection of occult metastases. In particular, imaging of the brain may be indicated for the exclusion of brain metastases in patients with clinically resectable, locally advanced NSCLC with nonsquamous histology [77]. The 2003 American Society of Clinical Oncology (ASCO) recommendations are that asymptomatic patients with Stage III disease being considered for aggressive local therapy (either surgery or radiation) should have CT or MR imaging performed [78]. MR imaging is more sensitive than CT and can detect smaller lesions [75]. Although MR can detect more lesions in a single patient, it has not been shown to upstage a greater number of patients compared with CT [79]. Consequently, the detection of smaller metastases by MRI is rarely of clinical significance.

Bone Metastases

Metastastic spread to the bones is evident in less than 10% of patients with NSCLC at the time of diagnosis [80, 40]. Patients with skeletal metastases are usually symptomatic or have laboratory abnormalities suggestive of bone metastases. Radionuclide bone scanning with 99Tc-MDP is usually performed to further evaluate a history of focal bone pain or elevated alkaline phosphatase. Because the detection of occult skeletal metastases by radionuclide 99Tc-MDP is low with a high false-positive rate, it is generally recommended that bone scintigraphy should not be routinely performed in asymptomatic patients [58]. However, this recommendation does not address the role of PET imaging in the detection of osseous metastases in patients with NSCLC. PET has been reported to reduce the number of false-negative and positive findings and to be more accurate than 99Tc-MDP bone scans in detecting skeletal metastases [81, 82]

Conclusion

Currently, CT is the workhorse of radiological tests in the staging of most patients with NSCLC. MR imaging has superior soft-tissue contrast resolution and, before the advent of MDCT, has been the preferred modality for the assessment of superior sulcus tumours. MR may also be useful in evaluating suspected pericardial or cardiac involvement. Whole body PET imaging is an integral component of NSCLC staging as it improves the detection of nodal and distant metastases and frequently alters patient management. Recently, integrated PET-CT scanners have been introduced allowing the acquisition of co-registered, spatially matched functional and morphological data. The staging of NSCLC has been reported to be more accurate with integrated PET-CT than when using visual correlation of PET and CT images performed separately. Accordingly, as the technique becomes more widely available, integrated PET-CT has the potential to be the imaging modality of choice for the staging of NSCLC.

REFERENCES

1. Mountain, C. F. (1997). Revisions in the International System for Staging Lung Cancer. *Chest*, **111**(6), 1710−17.

2. Park, B. J., Louie, O., Altorki, N. (2000). Staging and the surgical management of lung cancer. *Radiol Clin North Am*, **38**(3), 545−61.

3. Naruke, T., Tsuchiya, R., Kondo, H., *et al.* (2001). Prognosis and survival after resection for bronchogenic carcinoma based on the 1997 TNM-staging classification: the Japanese experience. *Ann Thorac Surg*, **71**(6), 1759−64.

4. Simon, G. R., Wagner, H. (2003). Small cell lung cancer. *Chest*, **123**(1 Suppl), 259S−271S.

5. Onitsuka, H., Tsukuda, M., Araki, A. *et al.* (1991). Differentiation of central lung tumor from postobstructive lobar collapse by rapid sequence computed tomography. *J Thorac Imaging*, **6**(2), 28−31.

6. Bourgouin, P. M., McLoud, T. C., Fitzgibbon, J. F., *et al.* (1991). Differentiation of bronchogenic carcinoma from postobstructive pneumonitis by magnetic resonance imaging: histopathologic correlation. *J Thorac Imaging*, **6**(2), 22−7.

7. Haramati, L. B., White, C. S. (2000). MR imaging of lung cancer. *Magn Reson Imaging Clin N Am*, **8**(1), 43−57.

8. Epstein, D. M., Stephenson, L. W., Gefter, W. B., *et al.* (1986). Value of CT in the preoperative assessment of lung cancer: a survey of thoracic surgeons. *Radiology*, **161**(2), 423−7.

9. Lahde, S., Paivansalo, M., Rainio, P. (1991). CT for predicting the resectability of lung cancer. A prospective study. *Acta Radiol*, **32**(6), 449−54.

10. Lewis, J. W., Jr., Pearlberg, J. L., Beute, G. H., *et al.* (1990). Can computed tomography of the chest stage lung cancer? Yes and no. *Ann Thorac Surg*, **49**(4), 591−5.

11. Quint, L. E., Glazer, G. M., Orringer, M. B. (1987). Central lung masses: prediction with CT of need for pneumonectomy versus lobectomy. *Radiology*, **165**(3), 735−8.

12. Galetta, D., Cesario, A., Margaritora, S., *et al.* (2003). Enduring challenge in the treatment of nonsmall cell lung cancer with clinical stage IIIB: results of a trimodality approach. *Ann Thorac Surg*, **76**(6), 1802−8.

13. Ichinose, Y., Fukuyama, Y., Asoh, H., *et al.* (2003). Induction chemoradiotherapy and surgical resection for selected stage IIIB non-small-cell lung cancer. *Ann Thorac Surg*, **76**(6), 1810−4.

14. Burnett, R. J., Wood, D. E. (1999). The new lung cancer staging system: what does it mean? *Surg Oncol Clin N Am*, **8**(2), 231−44.

15. Leong, S. S., Rocha Lima, C. M., Sherman, C. A., *et al.* (1999). The 1997 International Staging System for non-small cell lung cancer: have all the issues been addressed? *Chest*, **115**(1), 242−8.

16. Glazer, H. S., Kaiser, L. R., Anderson, D. J., *et al.* (1989). Indeterminate mediastinal invasion in bronchogenic carcinoma: CT evaluation. *Radiology*, **173**, 37−42.

17. Higashino, T., Ohno, Y., Takenaka, D., *et al.* (2005). Thin-section multiplanar reformats from multidetector-row CT data: utility for assessment of regional tumor extent in non-small cell lung cancer. *Eur J Radiol*, **56**(1), 48−55.

18. Lawler, L. P., Fishman, E. K. (2001). Multi-detector row CT of thoracic disease with emphasis on 3D volume rendering and CT angiography. *RadioGraphics*, **21**, 1257−73.

19. Boiselle, P. M. (2004). Staging of lung cancer with MDCT. In: U. J. Schoepf editor. Multi-detector Row CT of the Thorax. *Berlin Heidelberg: Springer-Verlag*, 205−14.

20. Musset, D., Grenier, P., Carette, M. F., *et al.* (1986). Primary lung cancer staging: prospective comparative study of MR imaging with CT. *Radiology*, **160**(3), 607−11.

21. Stiglbauer, R., Schurawitzki, H., Klepetko, W., *et al.* (1991). Contrast-enhanced MRI for the staging of bronchogenic carcinoma: comparison with CT and histopathologic staging− preliminary results. *Clin Radiol*, **44**(5), 293−8.

22. Mayr, B., Lenhard, M., Fink, U., *et al.* (1992). Preoperative evaluation of bronchogenic carcinoma: value of MR in T- and N-staging. *Eur J Radiol*, **14**(3), 245−51.

23. Ohno, Y., Sugimura, K., Hatabu, H. (2002). MR imaging of lung cancer. *Eur J Radiol*, **44**(3), 172−81.

24. White, C. S. (1996). MR evaluation of the pericardium and cardiac malignancies. *Magn Reson Imaging Clin N Am*, **4**(2), 237–51.

25. Seo, J. S., Kim, Y. J., Choi, B. W., *et al.* (2005). Usefulness of magnetic resonance imaging for evaluation of cardiovascular invasion: evaluation of sliding motion between thoracic mass and adjacent structures on cine MR images. *J Magn Reson Imaging*, **22**(2), 234–41.

26. Mountain, C. F., Dresler, C. M. (1997). Regional lymph node classification for lung cancer staging. *Chest*, **111**(6), 1718–23.

27. Andre, F., Grunenwald, D., Pignon, J. P., *et al.* (2000). Survival of patients with resected N2 non-small-cell lung cancer: evidence for a subclassification and implications. *J Clin Oncol*, **18**(16), 2981–9.

28. Toloza, E. M., Harpole, L., McCrory, D. C. (2003). Noninvasive staging of non-small cell lung cancer: a review of the current evidence. *Chest*, **123**(1 Suppl), 137S–146S.

29. Buy, J. N., Ghossain, M. A., Poirson, F., *et al.* (1988). Computed tomography of mediastinal lymph nodes in nonsmall cell lung cancer. A new approach based on the lymphatic pathway of tumor spread. *J Comput Assist Tomogr*, **12**(4), 545–52.

30. Glazer, G. M., Orringer, M. B., Chenevert, T. L., *et al.* (1988). Mediastinal lymph nodes: relaxation time/pathologic correlation and implications in staging of lung cancer with MR imaging. *Radiology*, **168**, 429–31.

31. Anzai, Y., Blackwell, K. E., Hirschowitz, S. L., *et al.* (1994). Initial clinical experience with dextran-coated superparamagnetic iron oxide for detection of lymph node metastases in patients with head and neck cancer. *Radiology*, **192**(3), 709–15.

32. Bellin, M. F., Beigelman, C., Precetti-Morel, S. (2000). Iron oxide-enhanced MR lymphography: initial experience. *Eur J Radiol*, **34**(3), 257–64.

33. Wiersema, M., Edell, E., Midthun, D. (2002). Prospective comparison of transbronchial needle aspirate (TBNA) and endosonography gioded biopsy (EUS-FNA) of mediastinal lymph nodes in patients with known or suspected nonsmall cell lung cancer. *Gastrointest. Endosc.*, **55**, 115.

34. Fritscher-Ravens, A., Davidson, B. L., Hauber, H. P., *et al.* (2003). Endoscopic ultrasound, positron emission tomography, and computerized tomography for lung cancer. *Am J Respir Crit Care Med*, **168**(11), 1293–7.

35. Eloubeidi, M. A., Cerfolio, R. J., Chen, V. K., *et al.* (2005). Endoscopic ultrasound-guided fine needle aspiration of mediastinal lymph node in patients with suspected lung cancer after positron emission tomography and computed tomography scans. *Ann Thorac Surg*, **79**(1), 263–8.

36. Rintoul, R. C., Skwarski, K. M., Murchison, J. T., *et al.* (2005). Endobronchial and endoscopic ultrasound-guided real-time fine-needle aspiration for mediastinal staging. *Eur Respir J*, **25**(3), 416–21.

37. Wallace, M. B., Silvestri, G. A., Sahai, A. V., *et al.* (2001). Endoscopic ultrasound-guided fine needle aspiration for staging patients with carcinoma of the lung. *Ann Thorac Surg*, **72**(6), 1861–7.

38. LeBlanc, J., Devereaux, B. M., Imperiale, T. F., *et al.* (2004). Endoscopic Ultrasound in Non-Small Cell Lung Cancer and Negative Mediastinum on Computed Tomography. *Am J Respir Crit Care Med*, **171**, 177–82.

39. Silvestri, G. A., Hoffman, B., Reed, C. E. (2003). One from column A: choosing between CT, positron emission tomography, endoscopic ultrasound with fine-needle aspiration, transbronchial needle aspiration, thoracoscopy, mediastinoscopy, and mediastinotomy for staging lung cancer. *Chest*, **123**(2), 333–5.

40. Quint, L. E., Tummala, S., Brisson, L. J., *et al.* (1996). Distribution of distant metastases from newly diagnosed non-small cell lung cancer. *Ann Thorac Surg*, **62**(1), 246–50.

41. Ratto, G. B., Piacenza, G., Frola, C., *et al.* (1991). Chest wall involvement by lung cancer: computed tomographic detection and results of operation. *Ann Thorac Surg*, **51**(2), 182–8.

42. Scott, I. R., Muller, N. L., Miller, R. R., *et al.* (1988). Resectable stage III lung cancer: CT, surgical, and pathologic correlation. *Radiology*, **166**(1 Pt 1), 75–9.

43. Pennes, D. R., Glazer, G. M., Wimbish, K. J., *et al.* (1985). Chest wall invasion by lung cancer: limitations of CT evaluation. *AJR Am J Roentgenol*, **144**(3), 507–11.

44. Glazer, H. S., Duncan-Meyer, J., Aronberg, D. J., *et al.* (1985). Pleural and chest wall invasion in bronchogenic carcinoma: CT evaluation. *Radiology*, **157**(1), 191–4.

45. Pearlberg, J. L., Sandler, M. A., Beute, G. H., *et al.* (1987). Limitations of CT in evaluation of neoplasms involving chest wall. *J Comput Assist Tomogr*, **11**(2), 290–3.

46. Murata, K., Takahashi, M., Mori, M., *et al.* (1994). Chest wall and mediastinal invasion by lung cancer: evaluation with multisection expiratory dynamic CT. *Radiology*, **191**(1), 251–5.

47. Sakai, S., Murayama, S., Murakami, J., *et al.* (1997). Bronchogenic carcinoma invasion of the chest wall: evaluation with dynamic cine MRI during breathing. *J Comput Assist Tomogr*, **21**(4), 595–600.

48. Johnson, D. H., Hainsworth, J. D., Greco, F. A. (1982). Pancoast's syndrome and small cell lung cancer. *Chest*, **82**(5), 602–6.

49. Paulson, D. L. (1975). Carcinomas in the superior pulmonary sulcus. *J Thorac Cardiovasc Surg*, **70**(6), 1095–104.

50. Detterbeck, F. C., Jones, D. R., Kernstine, K. H., *et al.* (2003). Lung cancer. Special treatment issues. *Chest*, **123**(1 Suppl), 244S–258S.

51. O'Connell, R. S., McLoud, T. C., Wilkins, E. W. (1983). Superior sulcus tumor: radiographic diagnosis and workup. *AJR Am J Roentgenol*, **140**(1), 25–30.

52. Webb, W. R., Gatsonis, C., Zerhouni, E. A., *et al.* (1991). CT and MR imaging in staging non-small cell bronchogenic carcinoma: report of the Radiologic Diagnostic Oncology Group. *Radiology*, **178**(3), 705–13.

53. Gefter, W. B. (1990). Magnetic resonance imaging in the evaluation of lung cancer. *Semin Roentgenol*, **25**(1), 73–84.

54. Heelan, R. T., Demas, B. E., Caravelli, J. F., *et al.* (1989). Superior sulcus tumors: CT and MR imaging. *Radiology*, **170**, 637–41.

55. McLoud, T. C., Filion, R. B., Edelman, R. R., *et al.* (1989). MR imaging of superior sulcus carcinoma. *J Comput Assist Tomogr*, **13**, 233–9.

56. Muers, M. F. (1994). Preoperative screening for metastases in lung cancer. *Thorax*, **49**(1), 1–2.

57. Tanaka, K., Kubota, K., Kodama, T., *et al.* (1999). Extrathoracic staging is not necessary for non-small-cell lung cancer with clinical stage T1–2 N0. *Ann Thorac Surg*, **68**(3), 1039–42.

58. Silvestri, G. A., Littenberg, B., Colice, G. L. (1995). The clinical evaluation for detecting metastatic lung cancer. A meta-analysis. *Am J Respir Crit Care Med*, **152**(1), 225–30.

59. Reed, C. E., Harpole, D. H., Posther, K. E., *et al.* (2003). Results of the American College of Surgeons Oncology Group Z0050 trial: the utility of positron emission tomography in staging potentially operable non-small cell lung cancer. *J Thorac Cardiovasc Surg*, **126**(6), 1943–51.

60. Oliver, T. W., Jr, Bernardino, M. E., Miller, J. I., *et al.* (1984). Isolated adrenal masses in nonsmall-cell bronchogenic carcinoma. *Radiology*, **153**(1), 217–8.

61. Pagani, J. J. (1984). Non-small cell lung carcinoma adrenal metastases. Computed tomography and percutaneous needle biopsy in their diagnosis. *Cancer*, **53**(5), 1058–60.

62. Pagani, J. J. (1983). Normal adrenal glands in small cell lung carcinoma: CT-guided biopsy. *AJR Am J Roentgenol*, **140**(5), 949–51.

63. Boland, G. W., Lee, M. J., Gazelle, G. S., *et al.* (1998). Characterization of adrenal masses using unenhanced CT: an analysis of the CT literature. *AJR Am J Roentgenol*, **171**(1), 201–4.

64. Pena, C. S., Boland, G. W., Hahn, P. F., *et al.* (2000). Characterization of indeterminate (lipid-poor) adrenal masses: use of washout characteristics at contrast-enhanced CT. *Radiology*, **217**(3), 798–802.

65. Boland, G. W., Hahn, P. F., Pena, C., *et al.* (1997). Adrenal masses: characterization with delayed contrast-enhanced CT. *Radiology*, **202**(3), 693–6.

66. Korobkin, M., Lombardi, T. J., Aisen, A. M., *et al.* (1995). Characterization of adrenal masses with chemical shift and gadolinium-enhanced MR imaging. *Radiology*, **197**(2), 411–18.

67. Baker, M. E., Pelley, R. (1995). Hepatic metastases: basic principles and implications for radiologists. *Radiology*, **197**(2), 329–37.

68. Hillers, T. K., Sauve, M. D., Guyatt, G. H. (1994). Analysis of published studies on the detection of extrathoracic metastases in patients presumed to have operable non-small cell lung cancer. *Thorax*, **49**(1), 14–19.

69. del Frate, C., Bazzocchi, M., Mortele, K. J., *et al.* (2002). Detection of liver metastases: comparison of gadobenate dimeglumine-enhanced and ferumoxides-enhanced MR imaging examinations. *Radiology*, **225**(3), 766–72.

70. Earnest, F., Ryu, J. H., Miller, G. M., *et al.* (1999). Suspected non-small cell lung cancer: incidence of occult brain and skeletal metastases and effectiveness of imaging for detection–pilot study. *Radiology*, **211**(1), 137–45.

71. Patchell, R. A., Tibbs, P. A., Walsh, J. W., *et al.* (1990). A randomized trial of surgery in the treatment of single metastases to the brain. *N Engl J Med*, **322**(8), 494–500.

72. Colice, G. L., Birkmeyer, J. D., Black, W. C., *et al.* (1995). Cost-effectiveness of head CT in patients with lung cancer without clinical evidence of metastases. *Chest*, **108**(5), 1264–71.

73. Figlin, R. A., Piantadosi, S., Feld, R. (1988). Intracranial recurrence of carcinoma after complete surgical resection of stage I, II, and III non-small-cell lung cancer. *N Engl J Med*, **318**(20), 1300–5.

74. Robnett, T. J., Machtay, M., Stevenson, J. P., *et al.* (2001). Factors affecting the risk of brain metastases after definitive chemoradiation for locally advanced non-small-cell lung carcinoma. *J Clin Oncol*, **19**(5), 1344–9.

75. Yokoi, K., Kamiya, N., Matsuguma, H., *et al.* (1999). Detection of brain metastasis in potentially operable non-small cell lung cancer: a comparison of CT and MRI. *Chest*, **115**(3), 714–9.

76. Pretreatment evaluation of non-small-cell lung cancer. The American Thoracic Society and The European Respiratory Society. (1997). *Am J Respir Crit Care Med*, **156**(1), 320–32.

77. Erasmus, J. J., Truong, M. T., Munden, R. F. (2005). CT, MR, and PET imaging in staging of non-small-cell lung cancer. *Semin Roentgenol*, **40**(2), 126–42.

78. Pfister, D. G., Johnson, D. H., Azzoli, C. G., *et al.* (2004). American Society of Clinical Oncology treatment of unresectable non-small-cell lung cancer guideline: update 2003. *J Clin Oncol*, **22**(2), 330–53.

79. Davis, P. C., Hudgins, P. A., Peterman, S. B., *et al.* (1991). Diagnosis of cerebral metastases: double-dose delayed CT vs contrast-enhanced MR imaging. *AJNR Am J Neuroradiol*, **12**(2), 293–300.

80. Ichinose, Y., Hara, N., Ohta, M., *et al.* (1989). Preoperative examination to detect distant metastasis is not advocated for asymptomatic patients with stages 1 and 2 non-small cell lung cancer. Preoperative examination for lung cancer. *Chest*, **96**(5), 1104–09.

81. Bury, T., Barreto, A., Daenen, F., *et al.* (1998). Fluorine-18 deoxyglucose positron emission tomography for the detection of bone metastases in patients with non-small cell lung cancer. *Eur J Nucl Med*, **25**(9), 1244–7.

82. Hsia, T. C., Shen, Y. Y., Yen, R. F., *et al.* (2002). Comparing whole body 18F-2-deoxyglucose positron emission tomography and technetium-99m methylene diophosphate bone scan to detect bone metastases in patients with non-small cell lung cancer. *Neoplasma*, **49**(4), 267–71.

83. The Guideline Development Group. The Diagnosis and Treatment of Lung Cancer. (2005). 12–13. The National Institute of Clinical Excellence.

84. Pass, H. I. (2005). Mediastinal staging 2005: pictures, scopes, and scalpels. *Semin Oncol*, **32**(3), 269–78.

Recommendations/Guidelines

National Institute for Clinical Excellence – NICE [83].
- In the assessment of mediastinal and chest wall invasion:
  CT alone cannot be relied upon
  Surgical assessment may be necessary if there are no other contraindications to resection.
- MRI should not be routinely be performed to assess T-stage in NSCLC, but should be considered for patients with superior sulcus tumours where necessary, to assess the extent of disease.
- Patients who are staged as candidates for surgery on CT should have a PET scan to look for involved intrathoracic lymph nodes and distant metastases.
- Patients who are otherwise surgical candidates and have on CT limited (1–2 stations) N2 disease of uncertain pathological significance should have a PET scan.
- Patients staged as N0 or N1 and MO (stages I and II) by CT and PET who are suitable for surgery should be offered surgical resection.
- Histological/cytological investigation should be performed to confirm N2/3 disease where PET is positive unless there is definite distant metastatic disease identified or there is high certainty that the N2/N3 disease is metastatic, for example, if there is a chain of high FDG uptake in lymph nodes.
- When a PET scan for N2/N3 disease is negative, biopsy is not required even if the patient's nodes are enlarged on CT.
- If PET is not available, suspected N2/N3 disease, as shown by CT (nodes with a short axis diameter of >1 cm), should be histologically sampled in patients being considered for surgical or radical radiotherapy.
- A CT or MRI should be performed in those patients with clinical signs or symptoms of brain metastasis.
- A bone scan should be performed for patients with localised signs or symptoms of bone metastases.

6

Positron Emission Tomography in Lung Cancer

Thomas B. Lynch and Gary J. R. Cook

Department of Nuclear Medicine and PET, Royal Marsden Hospital, Sutton, UK

Introduction

PET is a nuclear medicine imaging technique which, following injection of a positron emitting radiopharmaceutical, results in functional tomographic images. PET shares the advantages of nuclear medicine imaging over other radiological techniques including the ability to map function/metabolism before alterations in structure. In addition, some of the disadvantages of conventional nuclear medicine are overcome, in that spatial resolution of images is much improved and tomographic imaging is routine rather than an additional acquisition. Another advantage of PET is that it is relatively easy to measure and correct for the attenuation of photons that leave the body. This means that it is possible to measure radioactive concentrations accurately within tissues and, if necessary, express physiological processes in absolute units. The most widely used and computationally simple method of quantitation in clinical PET is the standardized uptake value (SUV). This is a semiquantitative index that measures the concentration of tracer within a tumour compared to the injected dose and is normalized to body weight. It has the potential to be an index of tracer uptake that can be compared between patients and at different time periods within the same patient and is commonly quoted in clinical PET publications.

PET has advanced in the last 15 years from being primarily a research tool to being an imaging modality with a number of clinical applications. With a relatively simple change in scanner design to allow whole body imaging and more recently with the development of combined PET/CT scanners, there has been a large growth in oncological applications where there is an increasing body of evidence that additional information can be gained over conventional imaging techniques that affects patient management whilst remaining cost-effective.

The role of clinical PET in oncology tends to be quite specific and does not necessarily replace conventional functional or anatomical imaging. Often, it offers a complementary procedure for supplying functional and metabolic information in the light of structural change. The structural/functional relationship can be further enhanced by combined PET/CT scanners that allow consecutive acquisition of PET and CT data whilst the patient is within the same scanner so that the anatomical and functional data can be accurately superimposed with the potential to improve diagnostic potential compared to PET alone (Fig. 6.1). PET is able to take advantage of some of the biologically important elements that have positron emitting isotopes such as carbon, nitrogen and oxygen. This means that organic compounds can be labelled by substitution with a radionuclide element without disturbance of normal biological pathways for the resultant molecule. PET tracers tend to have short half-lives compared to other radiopharmaceuticals used in nuclear medicine. As most PET radionuclides are produced in a cyclotron this has to be on-site for the

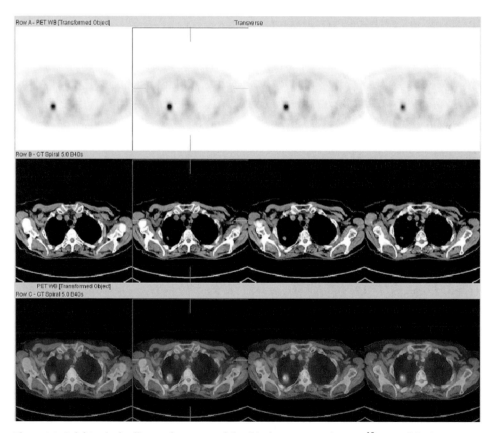

Figure 6.1 A right apical solitary pulmonary nodule. This demonstrates intense [18]FDG activity (SUV = 5.6) and was subsequently found to represent a squamous cell carcinoma (for a colour version of this figure please see the colour plate section)

shorter lived tracers. However, the most commonly used radiopharmaceutical, ^{18}fluoro-2-deoxy-D-glucose (^{18}FDG), has a half-life of approximately 110 minutes, a long enough time to allow transport between distant sites.

It has been recognized for many years that most malignant tumours exhibit increased glycolysis compared to normal tissues [1] and it is this property that is exploited in oncological PET imaging with ^{18}FDG which behaves as an analogue of glucose. Unlike glucose, ^{18}FDG does not enter further enzymatic reactions after conversion to ^{18}FDG-6-phosphate by hexokinase and being negatively charged, remains trapped in cells, allowing imaging to take place. A number of tumours have also been shown to overexpress glucose membrane transporters, identifying the mechanism by which increased amounts of ^{18}FDG are taken up into malignant cells. Of course, increased glycolysis is not specific to cancer cells but in most clinical situations the degree of uptake allows qualitative or quantitative differentiation of benign from malignant tissue.

It is in the investigation of lung cancer that ^{18}FDG-PET has gained the most robust evidence for its use in a clinical setting. The most validated clinical applications are the evaluation of indeterminate solitary pulmonary nodules and in the staging of non-small cell lung cancer before radical treatment with curative intent. However, other useful applications exist including assessing response to chemotherapy and radiotherapy, detecting recurrent disease and aiding radiotherapy planning.

Indeterminate Solitary Pulmonary Nodules

^{18}FDG PET has proved highly sensitive in the detection of cancer in pulmonary nodules with an average sensitivity of greater than 95% being reported [2] (Figs 6.1 and 6.2). The few false negatives are usually due to lesions that are too small for the abnormal metabolic activity to be adequately resolved (e.g. <1 cm) or a few cancers that only show relatively low metabolic activity (e.g. bronchioalveolar cell carcinoma [3]). The average specificity is less good, being reported at approximately 80% [2]. This is largely due to a number of benign active processes that accumulate ^{18}FDG. The proportion of false positives will probably vary geographically but a number of granulomatous processes, including histoplasmosis, tuberculosis and sarcoidosis can all show high uptake. In general the increased uptake within a pulmonary nodule can be assessed in two ways, either visually, by comparing the intensity of the nodule with the background blood pool activity or by means

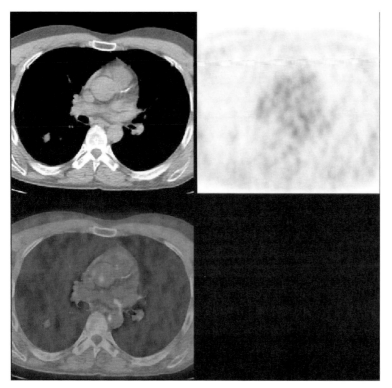

Figure 6.2 A right lower lobe nodule that does not demonstrate [18]FDG activity and is therefore likely to be benign (for a colour version of this figure please see the colour plate section)

of an SUV measurement. Attempts have been made to improve differentiation between benign and malignant processes by quantifying uptake with the calculation of the SUV [4]. An SUV = 2.5 is most frequently used as cut-off to maximally differentiate between malignant and benign nodules but others have found a non-quantitative approach sufficient. In view of the frequency of false positives, there will always be some inaccuracy in whatever method is used but with relatively few false negatives in lesions of a sufficient size, a negative scan can give confidence to follow-up patients non-invasively. This can be especially useful if biopsy has failed or if a biopsy is considered hazardous or technically difficult [5].

Staging Non-small Cell Lung Cancer

A number of retrospective trials have shown superior diagnostic accuracy of [18]FDG PET compared to conventional non-invasive staging techniques. The first

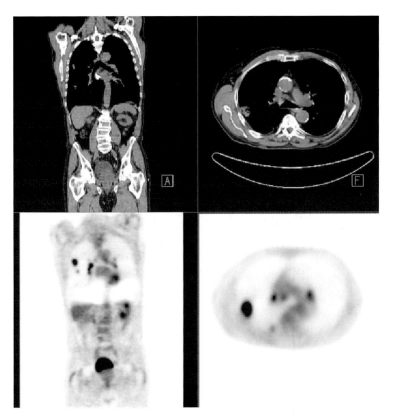

Figure 6.3 A right-sided peripheral carcinoma that found to ipsilateral hilar disease on CT staging.
[18]FDG PET confirms contralateral hilar disease

prospective trial of 102 patients comparing [18]FDG PET with conventional staging confirmed these findings, resulting in a different stage from the one determined by standard methods in 62 patients (42 upstaged and 20 downstaged) [6]. Mediastinal comparison was made to histology obtained at mediastinoscopy or thoracotomy and distant metastases were confirmed by additional imaging or biopsy. The sensitivity, specificity and accuracy for mediastinal staging were 91%, 86%, 87% for PET and 75%, 66%, 69% for CT (Fig. 6.3). In 11 out of 102 patients [18]FDG PET revealed distant metastatic disease (Figs 6.4 and 6.5). A subsequent prospective randomized study aimed to assess the effect of [18]FDG PET in avoiding futile thoracotomies (benign disease, explorative thoracotomy, IIIA-N2/IIIB, relapse or death within 12 months) [7]. In the group who underwent conventional workup preoperatively 41% had a futile thoracotomy whilst in the group where [18]FDG PET was included, only 21% had a futile thoracotomy giving a relative reduction of 51%. It was concluded that the addition of [18]FDG PET to

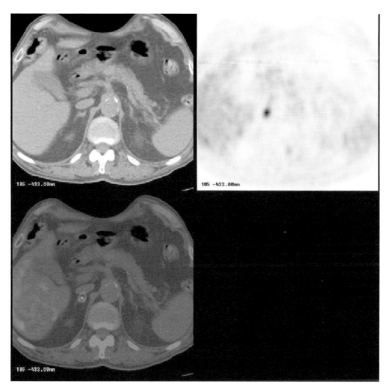

Figure 6.4 A small volume right adrenal metastasis that had not been suspected on the CT appearances but demonstrates abnormal activity on the PET scan

conventional workup prevented unnecessary surgery in 20% of patients with suspected non-small cell lung cancer.

Although accurate local staging is crucial for appropriate management of patients with lung cancer, it is the detection of distant metastatic disease that potentially impacts most on subsequent management as this almost always infers a palliative rather than curative approach. A number of studies have demonstrated that approximately 10% of patients will have distant metastases detected with PET that were unsuspected on conventional workup [6, 8]. Apart from the brain, where metastases may be inconspicuous against the normal high level of cortical activity, PET is otherwise a sensitive means of detecting small volume occult metastatic disease. PET is useful for differentiating adrenal metastases from benign incidental adrenal lesions [9] (Fig. 6.4) and is particularly sensitive in detecting skeletal metastases, being more sensitive than conventional bone scintigraphy [10] (Fig. 6.5).

These studies were performed before combined PET/CT scanners became available in 2001/2. A more recent study from one of the first institutions to use PET/CT

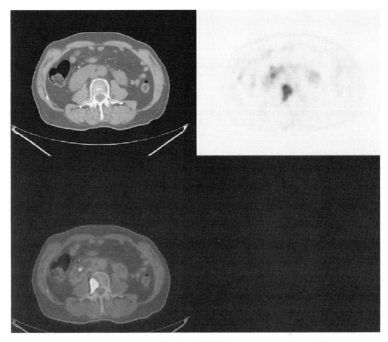

Figure 6.5 A previously undiagnosed vertebral bone metastasis identified by PET but with no abnormality seen on the CT component of the examination (for a colour version of this figure please see the colour plate section)

compared PET alone, CT, combined PET/CT and visual comparison of PET and CT side by side, in the staging of non-small cell lung cancer [11]. The study showed superiority for combined PET/CT over the other staging methods. The CT component of the PET/CT scans was performed without IV contrast and with a relatively low tube current (80 mA). It was in T staging where the most significant differences were seen (Fig. 6.6). [18]FDG PET on its own suffers from poor anatomical information, making it almost impossible to use this method for T staging. However, when combined with CT, these limitations are overcome and in this study PET/CT was statistically significantly better than all other methods. In addition, PET/CT showed more accurate N staging than PET alone and increased diagnostic certainty in two of the eight patients with distant metastases.

It is possible that the degree of [18]FDG activity may have prognostic importance. Dhital *et al.* noted that stage 1 lung cancers with an SUV of greater than 20 had a one year survival of only 17% compared to similar groups of stage 1 tumours with various levels of SUV of less than 20 who all had one year survival rates of greater than 60% [12].

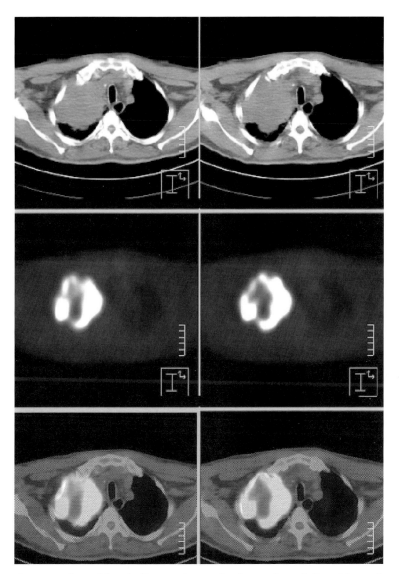

Figure 6.6 A large right apical lung carcinoma. The abnormal metabolic activity can be seen to extend into the chest wall anteriorly on the fused PET/CT images (for a colour version of this figure please see the colour plate section)

Assessing Response to Treatment

There are relatively few reports describing the use of ^{18}FDG PET in assessing treatment response but early publications have been encouraging. By measuring tumour metabolic activity it is anticipated that it may be possible to confirm effective treatment at an early stage before significant tumour shrinkage has occurred. This may enable an earlier change of treatment in those who are not responding and predict longer-term response and prognosis in those who do show metabolic response.

In a study of 47 patients with stage IIIA-N2 non-small cell lung cancer, [18]FDG PET was performed after 1 and 3 cycles of induction chemotherapy [13]. Residual [18]FDG activity after chemotherapy was the best prognostic factor and it was concluded that PET showed additional value over CT in monitoring response. In addition, it was found that relatively simple semiquantitative methods, e.g. SUV, performed as well as more complex kinetic analyses.

With regards to radiotherapy response, a small early study showed that those who showed a complete metabolic response remained locally controlled ($n = 4$) whilst those who showed only a partial response or no response had a 50% (4 of 8) mortality at two years [14]. Although uptake of [18]FDG due to inflammation in normal tissues related to radiotherapy could potentially obscure the measurement of response to radiotherapy, Hicks *et al.* found that this was not the case if a meticulous response assessment technique is used [15]. It was also noted that the inflammatory changes positively correlated with tumour response suggesting a link between tumour and normal tissue radiation sensitivity.

The same group evaluated [18]FDG PET in assessing response to radical radiotherapy/chemoradiotherapy in non-small cell lung cancer [16]. One year survival for those with a complete metabolic response was 93% compared to 47% in those who did not achieve a complete response. A complete metabolic response predicted a superior freedom from local and distant relapse.

Planning Radiotherapy

In addition, to the use of [18]FDG PET in the assessment of treatment response, there is an increasing vogue for using functional data in planning radiotherapy, particularly since the advent of combined PET/CT scanners. In one of the first studies to assess the impact of PET data on planning radiotherapy fields in the radical treatment of lung cancer it was found that 45 of 73 patients would have had treatment volumes changed if the PET data had been used for planning [17]. Some patients had fields increased to encompass PET positive nodes that had not been considered significant by conventional CT planning. In other patients it was possible to reduce the size of the field to the primary tumour when there was associated FDG-negative atelectasis (Fig. 6.7).

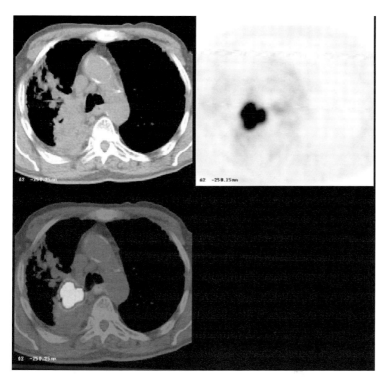

Figure 6.7 A right lower lobe carcinoma being considered for radiotherapy. On the CT it is difficult to determine the true extent of the tumour tissue and how much of the mass is due to benign collapse and consolidation. The PET images clearly show the anatomical boundaries between the benign and malignant tissue

Evaluation of Tumour Recurrence

In some patients in whom there is clinical suspicion of tumour relapse following therapy it can be difficult to differentiate post treatment changes from recurrent tumour with anatomical imaging techniques. It has been shown that [18]FDG PET can accurately differentiate benign post treatment fibrosis from recurrence [18]. When using a cut-off of an SUV of 2.5 the sensitivity for detecting recurrent tumour was 97% and specificity 100% in a series of 43 patients. Those with recurrence showed an average SUV of 7.6 compared to 1.6 in those with fibrosis only.

[18]FDG PET in Other Thoracic Malignancies

There are data to support the use of [18]FDG PET in other types of thoracic malignancy including small cell lung cancer and mesothelioma.

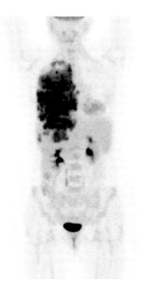

Figure 6.8 An extensive right-sided mesothelioma demonstrating intense FDG avidity

Small cell lung cancer is [18]FDG-avid and similar results have been reported with non-small cell lung cancer in regard to accuracy of staging, it being common for [18]FDG PET to upstage patients [19].

Most mesotheliomas are [18]FDG-avid (Fig. 6.8) but it has been reported that this method does not accurately define the local and nodal extent of disease but is helpful in detecting distant metastases [20] A potential problem in assessing mesothelioma is found in patients who have had a talc pleurodesis as this can cause a pleural reaction that accumulates [18]FDG for months or years after the procedure.

Diagnostic Issues and Pitfalls in [18]FDG PET Imaging

One of the commonest problems with [18]FDG PET imaging is due to the increased uptake by benign processes. This has been described above with respect to inde-terminate solitary nodules but remains a potential problem for other applications of this scanning method. To some extent the number of false positives has improved since the advent of PET/CT where the anatomical correlate can be helpful in correctly assigning FDG activity to tissues with benign characteristics. However, [18]FDG is not a tumour-specific tracer and there is always the need to be wary of these potential pitfalls. Another potential limitation for [18]FDG PET is that it is relatively insensitive in detecting brain metastases. This is primarily because

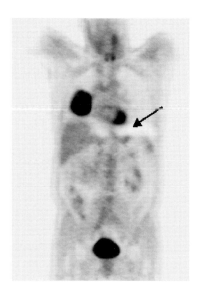

Figure 6.9 An attenuation correction artefact caused by differences in position of the diaphragm in the PET and CT components of the acquisition. This causes an apparent reduction in activity at the level of the diaphragm seen as a photon-deficient stripe (arrow)

normal brain cortex shows high uptake of [18]FDG often obscuring uptake in metastases. If brain metastases are suspected then MRI or CT should be used to evaluate rather than PET. Although combining PET and CT has reduced a number of potential pitfalls there are some artefacts that have been introduced by this technique [21]. The commonest is related to mis-registration of the two image data sets due to differences in patient or organ position between the two scan acquisitions.

CT and PET acquisitions are made sequentially in PET/CT systems, with the data sets acquired from the two parts of the gantry being intrinsically aligned and allowing accurate registration provided that there is no difference in position of organs between the two scans. CT images are often acquired during a single breath hold over the thorax whereas PET images are acquired during tidal breathing over 20–30 minutes and the resultant PET image represents an average position of the thoracic cage during this time. The use of CT for attenuation correction of the PET data can result in artefacts when there is mis-registration due to breathing differences. The most commonly encountered artefact is an apparent loss of counts in the corrected PET image at the level of the diaphragm (Fig. 6.9). Differences in breathing patterns between CT and PET scans may lead to mis-registration of pulmonary nodules particularly in the peripheral and basal lung regions where the differences may approach 15 mm [22]. It is also possible for objects just below the diaphragm (e.g. liver metastases) to appear in the lung bases on corrected PET images. Mis-registration artefacts can be minimized by performing the CT scan during normal relaxed expiration but it is likely that when accurate registration in the thorax is very important (e.g. radiotherapy planning for lung cancer), then respiratory gating techniques will be developed. Another factor to be considered is that the sensitivity for malignant nodules may be less in the lung due to respiratory motion than in other parts of the body. It is not uncommon to detect small subcentimetre pulmonary metastases on the CT component of PET/CT but to be unable to resolve increased [18]FDG activity.

Future Applications

Although it is likely that [18]FDG PET will remain the workhorse of clinical PET in oncology for many years, it may be presumed that new tracers will be developed to overcome some of the shortcomings in certain applications. There has been increasing interest in the use of ^{18}F-fluorothymidine ([18]FLT) to monitor tumour proliferation with the hope that there will more more specificity for malignancy than with [18]FDG. Whilst the specificity may be improved there may be a loss of sensitivity for detecting metastatic disease with [18]FLT suggesting that this tracer cannot take the place of [18]FDG for staging [23]. There is also interest in choline-based tracers that reflect tumour membrane turnover. There is early work that suggests it is possible to differentiate tuberculous lesions from malignant ones using ^{11}C-choline [24]. [18]FDG is taken up avidly by both processes but ^{11}C-choline appears more specific for malignant tissue.

Radiation oncologists have been interested in measuring tumour hypoxia for many years as this characteristic is known to confer resistance in tumours to radiotherapy and some forms of chemotherapy. However, non-invasive methods of measuring hypoxia have not been available. A number of PET tracers, including ^{18}F-fluormisonidazole, are selectively trapped in hypoxic tissue and have the potential to measure this aspect of tumour physiology allowing the administration of radiation sensitisers or to boost radiation dose to hypoxic tumour foci [25].

Conclusion

There is no doubt that [18]FDG PET or PET/CT has a significant role to play in optimal staging of patients with non-small cell lung cancer being considered for radical treatment. There is now sufficient evidence to recommend the routine use of PET in this regard. There is early evidence to suggest that there may also be roles for ^{18}FDG PET (and possibly newer tracers) at other stages in the management of patients with non-small cell lung cancer and other thoracic malignancies. With the advent of PET/CT it is possible that in the future a single PET/CT examination will be performed early in the course of a patient's management rather than as an additional examination at the end of routine staging procedures.

REFERENCES

1. Warburgh, O. (1954). On the origin of cancer cells. *Science*, **123**, 306−14.
2. Shon, I. H., O'Doherty, M. J., Maisey, M. N. (2002). Positron emission tomography in lung cancer. *Semin Nucl Med*, **32**, 240−71.
3. Higashi, K., Ueda, Y., Seki, H., *et al*. (1998). Fluorine-18-FDG PET imaging is negative in bronchioloalveolar lung carcinoma. *J Nucl Med*, **39**, 1016−20.
4. Lowe, V. J., Hoffman, J. M., DeLong, D. M., Patz, E. F., Coleman, R. E. (1994). Semiquantitative and visual analysis of FDG-PET images in pulmonary abnormalities. *J Nucl Med*, **35**, 1771−6.
5. Hain, S. F., Curran, K. M., Beggs, A. D., Fogelman, I., O'Doherty, M. J., Maisey, M. N. (2001). FDG-PET as a "metabolic biopsy" tool in thoracic lesions with indeterminate biopsy. *Eur J Nucl Med*, **28**, 1336−40.
6. Pieterman, R. M., van Putten, J. W., Meuzelaar, J. J., Mooyaart, E. L., Vaalburg, W., Koeter, G. H., Fidler, V., Pruim, J., Groen, H. J. (2000). Preoperative staging of non-small-cell lung cancer with positron-emission tomography. *N Engl J Med*, **343**, 254−61.
7. van Tinteren, H., Hoekstra, O. S., Smit, E. F., van den Bergh, J. H., *et al*. (2002). Effectiveness of positron emission tomography in the preoperative assessment of patients with suspected non-small-cell lung cancer: the PLUS multicentre randomised trial. *Lancet*, **359**, 1388−93.
8. Valk, P. E., Pounds, T. R., Hopkins, D. M., Haseman, M. K., *et al*. (1995). Staging non-small cell lung cancer by whole body positron emission tomography imaging. *Ann Thor Surg*, **60**, 1573−81.
9. Erasmus, J. J., Patz, E. F., McAdamas, H. P., Murray, J. G., *et al*. (1997). Evaluation of adrenal masses in patientys with bronchogenic carcinoma using 18F-fluorodeoxyglucose positron emission tomography. *Am J Roentgenol*, **168**, 1357−60.
10. Bury, T., Barreto, A., Daenen, F., Barthelemy, N., *et al*. (1998). Fluorine-18 deoxyglucose positron emission tomography for the detection of bone metastases in patients with non-small cell lung cancer. *Eur J Nucl Med*, **25**, 1244−47.
11. Lardinois, D., Weder, W., Hany, T. F., Kamel, E. M., *et al*. (2003). Staging of non-small-cell lung cancer with integrated positron-emission tomography and computed tomography. *N Engl J Med*, **348**, 2500−7.
12. Dhital, K., Saunders, C. A., Seed, P. T., O'Doherty, M. J., Dussek, J. (2000). 18FDG PET and its prognostic value in lung cancer. *Eur J Cardiothorac Surg*, **18**, 425−8.

13. Hoekstra, C. J., Stroobants, S. G., Smit, E. F., Vansteenkiste, J., *et al.* (2005). Prognostic relevance of response evaluation using 18F -2-fluoro-2-deoxy-D-glucose positron emission tomography in patients with locally advanced non-small-cell lung cancer. *J Clin Oncol*, **23**, 8362−70.

14. Hebert, M. E., Lowe, V. J., Hoffman, J. M., Patz, E. F., Anscher, M. S. (1996). Positron emission tomography in the pretreatment evaluation and follow-up of non-small cell lung cancer patients treated with radiotherapy: preliminary findings. *Am J Clin Oncol*, **19**, 416−21.

15. Hicks, R. J., Mac Manus, M. P., Matthews, J. P., Hogg, A., *et al.* (2004). Early FDG-PET imaging after radical radiotherapy for non-small-cell lung cancer: inflammatory changes in normal tissues correlate with tumor response and do not confound therapeutic response evaluation. *Int J Radiat Oncol Biol Phys*, **60**, 412−8.

16. Mac Manus, M. P., Hicks, R. J., Matthews, J. P., Wirth, A., *et al.* (2005). Metabolic (FDG-PET) response after radical radiotherapy/chemoradiotherapy for non-small cell lung cancer correlates with patterns of failure. *Lung Cancer*, **49**, 95−108.

17. Vanuytsel, L. J., Vansteenkiste, J. F., Stroobants, S. G., De Leyn, P. R., *et al.* (2000). The impact of (18)F-fluoro-2-deoxy-D-glucose positron emission tomography (FDG-PET) lymph node staging on the radiation treatment volumes in patients with non-small cell lung cancer. *Radiother Oncol*, **55**, 317−24.

18. Patz, E. F., Lowe, V. J., Hoffman, J. M., Paine, S. S., *et al.* (1994). Persistent or recurrent broncho-genic carcinoma: detection with PET and 2- F-18 -2-deoxy-D-glucose. *Radiology*, **191**, 379−82.

19. Bradley, J. D., Dehdashti, F., Mintun, M. A., Govindan, R., *et al.* (2004). Positron emission tomography in limited-stage small-cell lung cancer: a prospective study. *J Clin Oncol*, **22**, 3248−54.

20. Flores, R. M., Akhurst, T., Gonen, M., Larson, S. M., Rusch, V. W. (2003). Positron emission tomography defines metastatic disease but not locoregional disease in patients with malignant pleural mesothelioma. *J Thorac Cardiovasc Surg*, **126**, 11−16.

21. Cook, G. J., Wegner, E., Fogleman, I. (2004). Pitfalls and Artefacts in 18 FDG PET and PET/CT Oncologic imaging. *Semin Nucl Med*, **34**, 122−33.

22. Goerres, G. W., Kamel, E., Seifert, B., *et al.* (2002). Accuracy of image coregistration of pulmonary lesions in patients with non-small cell lung cancer using an integrated PET/CT system. *J Nucl Med*, **43**, 1469−75.

23. Buck, A. K., Hetzel, M., Schirrmeister, H., Halter, G., *et al.* (2005). Clinical relevance of imaging proliferative activity in lung nodules. *Eur J Nucl Med Mol Imaging*, **32**, 525−33.

24. Hara, T., Kosaka, N., Suzuki, T., Kudo, K., Niino, H. (2003). Uptake rates of 18F-fluorodeoxyglucose and 11C-choline in lung cancer and pulmonary tuberculosis: a positron emission tomography study. *Chest*, **124**, 893−901.

25. Eschmann, S. M., Paulsen, F., Reimold, M., Dittmann, H., *et al.* (2005). Prognostic impact of hypoxia imaging with 18F-misonidazole PET in non-small cell lung cancer and head and neck cancer before radiotherapy. *J Nucl Med*, **46**, 253−60.

7

Contemporary Issues in the Systemic Treatment of Lung Cancer

Alistair Ring and Joseph Prendiville

Guy's, King's and St Thomas' Cancer Centre, London, UK

Introduction

Lung cancer is conveniently divided into two major histopathological subtypes known as small cell lung cancer (SCLC) and non-small cell lung cancer, (NSCLC) by virtue of their very differing responses to chemotherapy. Since the introduction of systemic chemotherapy in the 1970s SCLC has been regarded as a highly chemosensitive tumour where chemotherapy can dramatically alter the natural course of the disease. In contrast NSCLC has been regarded as relatively resistant to cytotoxic chemotherapy. While most patients with SCLC continue to derive significant benefit from chemotherapy which always warrants its use, there has not been dramatic progress in further improving survival. This is in spite of much innovative research over the past two decades. In contrast over the same period of time, we have witnessed developments in the treatment of advanced-stage NSCLC where we have gone from a situation of uncertainty as to whether even first line chemotherapy was of any value at all, to now knowing that patients with advanced-stage disease gain survival advantage and improvements in quality of life from first, second and third line treatments. Patients with advanced NSCLC are also benefiting from treatment with novel biological therapies, though their exact role has yet to be completely defined. Furthermore, several trials have now also clearly documented the benefit to patients form adjuvant treatment following resection of early-stage NSCLC.

Non-small Cell Lung Cancer

Systemic chemotherapy has three potential roles in the management of patients with NSCLC: first, as palliative treatment of advanced disease (Stages 111B [with a pleural effusion] and IV [and MI]), second, in complementing radiotherapy for locally advanced disease (Stages IIIAN2 or IIIB [without a pleural effusion] and third, in complementing surgery for early-stage resectable disease (Stages I to IIIA [N1]) — the latter either post-operatively (termed adjuvant chemotherapy) or preoperatively (known as neo-adjuvant chemotherapy). This chapter will focus on palliative chemotherapy for advanced-stage disease and chemotherapy for early-stage disease (adjuvant or neo-adjuvant).

Palliative Chemotherapy for Advanced-stage NSCLC

Stage IIIB (with a pleural effusion) and IV NSCLC are generally regarded as incurable, with 5-year survival rates of less than 5%. Chemotherapy may be considered as a sole primary treatment modality in advanced stage disease or in combination with radiotherapy in locally advanced disease. In 1995 a large meta-analysis of randomized trials of cisplatin-based chemotherapy versus best supportive care indicated improvements in median survival of between one and two months [1]. Importantly, these modest improvements in overall survival appeared to be accompanied by significantly improved symptom control and quality of life [2−4]. Over recent years several newer generation agents have shown activity in advanced NSCLC. These drugs, which include gemcitabine, vinorelbine, docetaxel, paclitaxel and irinotecan, all demonstrate response rates in the region of 20% when given as single agents in first line treatment. However, when given in combination with platinums (either cisplatin or carboplatin) response rates of between 16 and 43% have been reported [5−13]. As a result, the National Institute for Health and Clinical Excellence (NICE) recommends that gemcitabine, paclitaxel and vinorelbine should each be considered as part of first line chemotherapy options for advanced-stage NSCLC patients [14]. The guidance also concludes that there is insufficient evidence on how these drugs compare with each other, and indeed where comparative studies have now become available there is no one combination that appears to be superior. Review of ECOG and SWOG phase III trials, as well as CALGB, TAX 326, NCCGS, and European trials, do not show a clear-cut superiority of any single regimen over the others [10, 15, 16].

In the chemotherapeutic treatment of advanced-stage NSCLC, it has been stated that 'there is a choice of treatments rather than a treatment of choice' [16]. Choice will therefore very often be based on familiarity with the chemotherapeutic regimen, expected toxicity, convenience of administration and costs. Physicians and patients may prefer taxol or taxotere with a platinum agent because these drugs may be given as a three-weekly regimen, not requiring a day-eight visit to hospital.

Those choosing gemcitabine with a platinum agent will be reassured by the substantive amount of data with this drug, and also by the recent meta-analysis demonstrating an improved time to relapse, though the trend to overall survival was not statistically significant [17]. Gemcitabine and platinum remains a regimen requiring both a day-one and a day-eight visit to hospital. There may be a preference for vinorelbine and a platinum agent because of the substantive amount of data with this drug and, more recently, the introduction of an oral formulation which transforms a day-one and day-eight regimen into a three-weekly regimen. Furthermore, the oral formulation of vinorelbine allows a completely non-intravenous regimen for elderly patients and those with poor performance status who may be best treated with a non-platinum single agent therapy (see below).

In an attempt to improve on the advantages of platinum third generation doublets as described above, combinations of two new agents with platinum in a triplet regimen have been investigated. However, these have yet to show a convincing survival advantage over platinum doublets and are more toxic. Therefore triplet platinum-based regimens have not, to date, been endorsed by NICE [14, 18]. Similarly, there do not seem to be significant differences in survival when combinations of two new non-platinum agents are compared with platinum-based treatments [14, 19]. However, such an approach may improve quality of life for patients on treatment, but many feel more randomized trials incorporating such analyses are needed before such combinations can be recommended and the extra expense justified.

For many years cisplatin has been the mainstay of chemotherapy for both NSCLC and SCLC. However carboplatin, an analogue of cisplatin has a more favourable toxicity profile (less nephrotoxicity, ototoxicity, neurotoxicity and emetogenesis) and can be administered with greater safety to patients with impaired renal function. Thus, the use of carboplatin extends the envelope of patients eligible for treatment with chemotherapy. However, a recent meta-analysis of eight randomized trials, which compared cisplatin with carboplatin regimens, showed that cisplatin-based treatments yielded higher response rates [20]. Moreover, in the five trials which compared the platinums in combination with a new agent (gemcitabine, paclitaxel or docetaxel), chemotherapy consisting of cisplatin with a new agent yielded 11% longer survival than carboplatin with the same new agent. Therefore, although carboplatin may be used to substitute for cisplatin on the basis of toxicity and convenience, it is not necessarily as effective. There is currently an on-going randomized National Cancer Research Institute (NCRI) trial being conducted in the United Kingdom with a three-arm design comparing a third-generation doublet with three different platinum arms: cisplatin $50 \, mg/m^2$; cisplatin $80 \, mg/m^2$; or carboplatin AUC 6 (Wright GFR estimation).

Despite treatment with carboplatin, many patients with advanced-stage NSCLC are unable to tolerate platinum-based chemotherapy. In such cases treatment with a single new agent is an option. Several studies have shown that gemcitabine, docetaxel and vinorelbine have activity as single agents and are well tolerated. In the ELVIS trial, elderly patients (70 years or older) with advanced NSCLC were randomized to receive vinorelbine ($30 \, mg/m^2$ on days 1 and 8, every three weeks) or best supportive care [3]. The study showed that there was a survival advantage of seven weeks in those receiving chemotherapy and that these patients reported fewer lung cancer-related symptoms and better quality of life functioning scales. Similar results have been reported for docetaxel compared with best supportive care [21] and it may be that in some patients, particularly the elderly or those with a poor performance status, single agent chemotherapy is an appropriate option. Vinorelbine offers the scheduling advantage of having an oral formulation and the patient convenience of no intravenous treatment.

As chemotherapy becomes more widely accepted as an option in advanced NSCLC and also in the treatment of earlier stage disease, the prospect of an increasing population of patients relapsing after first-line chemotherapy must be considered. In those patients who still have an acceptable performance status second-line chemotherapy may be an option. In one randomized trial, 204 patients with NSCLC previously treated with platinum-based chemotherapy were randomized to treatment with docetaxel ($75-100 \, mg/m^2$ every three weeks) or best supportive care [22]. In patients receiving $75 \, mg/m^2$ of docetaxel, there was a significant improvement in survival when compared to best supportive care (7.5 months versus 4.6 months; $p = 0.01$). Morevoer, all quality-of-life parameters favoured the chemotherapy arm, with the differences in pain and fatigue reaching statistical significance.

More recently a trial comparing second-line treatment with docetaxel together with the multi-targeted antifolate agent, pemetrexed has shown equivalent efficacy in response rates, progression-free and overall survival, but with a toxicity profile favouring pemetrexed [23]. Currently, taxotere is the only NICE-guided second-line drug for NSCLC in the United Kingdom. However, the situation may change when the data on pemetrexed (which is currently licensed for this indication) is reviewed. NICE may also sanction the use of erlotinib (a small molecule oral tyrosine kinase inhibitor) as second- or third-line treatment for NSCLC, as it has recently received a licence for this indication (see below under novel agents).

Adjuvant (Post-operative) Chemotherapy for Early-stage Disease

It is salutary to note that even survival in patients with apparently curative resections of NSCLC is still only approximately 40% at five years [24, 25]. Moreover, the incidence of recurrence in patients with early-stage resectable disease is as high as 70% in many studies. Chemotherapy given after complete resection of solid tumour (termed adjuvant chemotherapy), has been established practice for breast and bowel cancer for 15 years. A meta-analysis in 1995 suggested that adjuvant cisplatin-based chemotherapy may provide an absolute (although not statistically significant) survival advantage of 5% at five years [1]. Seven co-operative groups have since launched prospective trials, which have been reported (Table 7.1). Three of these trials provided negative results but all included 'old style' platinum regimens: ALPI [29], INT 0115 [30], and BLT [31]. However, four of the seven trials have provided encouraging results. One study, conducted by the International Adjuvant Lung Cancer Collaborative Group (IALT) is, to date, the largest adjuvant lung cancer trial reported [25]. The survival benefit seen with IALT was small (4.1% at five years; $p = 0.03$), but compares favourably with results which have historically been quoted to justify adjuvant chemotherapy in breast and colon cancer. In the three remaining trials with positive results, third-generation drug combinations were employed and have demonstrated spectacular results with improvements in survival at five years of 8% and 15% with the use of adjuvant vinorelbine and cisplatin [27, 28], and 12% at four years with adjuvant paclitaxel and carboplatin [26]. For the purpose of illustrating this excellent adjuvant effect, we have included a figure from the Winton study which is the trial with the most dramatic survival advantage at five years of 15% using vinorelbine and cisplatin (Fig. 7.1).

Many issues remain regarding the exact benefit in different stages of resected NSCLC. However, in a comprehensive review published in 2005, it was concluded that 'there is compelling evidence to now recommend adjuvant platinum-based combination chemotherapy for patients after resection of early-stage disease' [32].

In the discussion above we have referred to trials carried out in the western hemisphere. However, there are also promising Japanese data using adjuvant uracil-tegafur (UFT), an oral prodrug of 5-fluorouracil (5-FU), with or without cisplatin. One meta-analysis has put the benefit of adjuvant 5-FU in resected stage 1A NSCLC at 17% [33]. The problem is that 5-FU is not a drug associated with a significant benefit in advanced-stage disease, a sine qua non for any drug being considered for use in the setting of adjuvant therapy. Furthermore, while there is

Table 7.1. Trials investigating the role of post-operative adjuvant chemotherapy for non-small cell lung cancer

Trial (reference)	Disease stages	Chemotherapy	5-year overall survival *Experimental vs. Observation arm*	Comments
International Adjuvant Lung Trial (IALT) (25)	I–III	Cisplatin 80–120 mg/m² 3–4 cycles, together with vindesine 3 mg/m², vinblastine 4 mg/m², vinorelbine 30 mg/m² or etoposide 100 mg/m²	44.5 vs. 40.4% (p < 0.03)	
CALGB 9633 (26)	IB	Carboplatin AUC 6 and paclitaxel 200 mg/m² for 4 cycles	71% vs. 59% ($p = 0.03$)	Survival given at 4 years
JBR 10 (27)	IB, II	Vinorelbine 25 mg/m² weekly for 16 weeks and cisplatin 50 mg/m² days 1 and 8 every 4 weeks for 4 cycles.	69% vs. 54% ($p = 0.03$)	Result not significant for IB subgroup
ANITA (28)	IB, II, IIIA	Vinorelbine 30 mg/m² weekly for 16 weeks and cisplatin 100 mg/m² every 4 weeks for 4 cycles.	51% vs. 43% ($p = 0.01$)	Result not significant for IB subgroup
ALPI trial (29)	I,II,IIIA	Three cycles of mitomycin 8 mg/m² day 1, vindesine 3 mg/m² days 1 and 8, cisplatin 100 mg/m² day1. Once every three weeks.	Not given	No statistically significant difference in overall survival.

Table 7.1. (*cont.*)

Trial (reference)	Disease stages	Chemotherapy	5-year overall survival *Experimental vs. Observation arm*	Comments
INT 0115 (30)	II, IIIA	Four cycles of cisplatin 60 mg/m^2 and etoposide 120 mg/m^2 days 1–3, once every 4 weeks.	Not given	No statistically significant difference in overall survival. Postoperative radiotherapy given in both experimental and control arms.
BLT (31)	I,II,IIIA,IIIB,IV	Three cycles of cisplatin, with vindesine, mitomycin, ifosfamide or mitomycin, vinblastine, vinorelbine	74% vs. 60% (2 year, $p=0.90$)	No statistically significant difference in overall survival

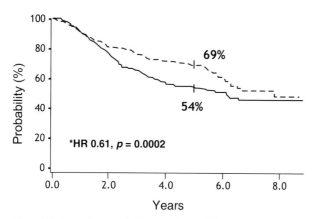

Figure 7.1 Overall survival of 482 patients with stages IB and II non-small cell lung cancer, enrolled in the JBR 10 study [27], according to treatment arm: observation alone (——) vs. adjuvant vinorelbine and cisplatin (– – –)

some evidence that the pharmacokinetics of tegafur is similar in Western and Japanese patients [34], it is not clear whether there is an unknown oncological pharmacodynamic effect.

Neo-adjuvant Chemotherapy (Pre-operative Chemotherapy) for Early-stage Disease

Neo-adjuvant chemotherapy is of proven value in the induction of both radiological and pathological response in resectable NSCLC. In a trial of patients with stage IB-IIIA disease there was a non-significant trend towards improved survival of 7% (59 vs. 52%) at two years when surgery was preceded by chemotherapy [35]. Similarly, in a recent North American study, there was a non-significant trend toward improvement in survival at two years of 6% when surgery was preceded by chemotherapy with carboplatin and paclitaxel [36]. Given these non-significant data for neo-adjuvant chemotherapy and the report of positive trials for adjuvant chemotherapy, the question arises as to whether neo-adjuvant chemotherapy is likely to offer any benefit over adjuvant therapy for the treatment of early-stage resectable NSCLC. In an attempt to address the issue, in the three-arm NATCH trial, patients with resectable NSCLC have been randomized either to surgery alone, pre-operative (i.e. neo-adjuvant) chemotherapy followed by surgery or surgery followed by post-operative (i.e. adjuvant) chemotherapy [37]. There is also consideration being given to a UK NCRI study of neoadjuvant versus adjuvant

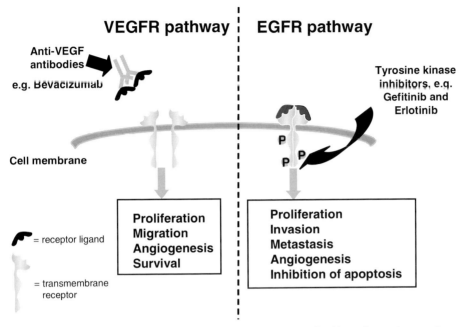

Figure 7.2 Vascular Endothelial Growth Factor Receptor (VEGFR) and Epidermal Growth Factor Receptor (EGFR) pathways involved in membrane signal transduction pathways in non-small cell lung cancer

chemotherapy. Until the results of such trials are declared, adjuvant chemotherapy with a third-generation platinum combination remains the standard treatment when for resectable (i.e. early-stage) NSCLC.

Novel Agents

In recent years significant advances have been made in our understanding of the molecular mechanisms that underlie malignant transformation of cells and tumour progression. In NSCLC it has become apparent that the epidermal growth factor receptor (EGFR) has a critical role in mediating tumour cell proliferation, angiogenesis and apoptosis. Therefore, agents which block the tyrosine kinase activity of the EGFR-receptor have been developed (Fig. 7.2). Two such drugs, gefitinib and erlotinib, (both orally active) are available for use. In the IDEAL trials 1 and 2, gefitinib was used to treat patients with advanced NSCLC who had previously received platinum-based chemotherapy [38, 39]. The objective tumour response rates were modest at 18% and 11%, respectively, but importantly symptomatic improvements were observed in 40% of patients. Unfortunately, no improvement in survival has been demonstrated when gefitinib or erlotinib are added to chemotherapy for advanced disease [40–42]. However, in a recent randomized placebo-controlled trial erlotinib was shown to improve survival (6.7 vs. 4.7 months, $p = 0.001$) and symptom control in patients with advanced NSCLC who had previously received at least one line of chemotherapy [43]. A further important observation has been that different active mutations in the EGFR may correlate which with sensitivity to gefitinib [44]. Thus, in addition to producing meaningful symptom and survival benefits in patients with NSCLC, there is the tantalizing prospect of identifying those patients most likely to respond to treatment.

Following the early successes of EGFR-targeted therapies in NSCLC, a large number of other novel targeted therapies have been explored. In the recent ECOG 4599 study, patients with stage IIIB/IV non-squamous NSCLC were treated with carboplatin and paclitaxel with or without the anti-vascular endothelial growth factor (VEGF) antibody, bevacizumab (Fig. 7.2). Patients who received bevacizumab had a higher response rate (27% vs. 10%, $p < 0.0001$), and overall survival (12.5 vs. 10.2 months, $p = 0.008$) [45]. This is the first time that the addition of a targeted agent to chemotherapy for NSCLC has been shown to improve survival and represents an exciting development in the evolution of this class of agents.

Other novel agents, which have also shown activity in phase I/II NSCLC, include the proteasome inhibitor bortezomib [46], anti-EGFR antibody cetuximab [47], and the farnesyl transferase inhibitor, tipifarnib [48]. The challenge now being faced is how best to integrate these drugs into clinical practice: the questions are whether such drugs should be used concurrently with chemotherapy or sequentially and what is the role of maintenance therapy and finally the economic considerations.

Small Cell Lung Cancer

Small cell lung cancer (SCLC) is a rapidly progressive malignancy which is usually a systemic disease at the outset. Consequently, surgery is inappropriate for the vast majority of patients. Patients with this subtype of lung cancer are conveniently staged as having either limited (LS-SCLC) stage, where disease is confined to one hemithorax but includes ipsilateral and contralateral supraclavicular lymphadenopathy or extensive (ES-SCLC) stage, in which tumour has spread outside the limited stage definition (e.g. to cervical nodes, the contralateral lung, liver, brain, adrenal glands). Before the introduction of systemic treatment with chemotherapy, the prognosis for SCLC was dreadful with median survival the order of six weeks for patients with ES-SCLC and three months for those with LS-SCLC. However, with the advent of combination chemotherapy in patients with ES-SCLC, median survival has been extended to around nine months. In LS-SCLC, chemotherapy combined with thoracic irradiation and (where indicated) prophylactic cranial irradiation extends median survival to approximately 18 months. Yet, in spite of this progress, data from the Surveillance, Epidemiology and End Results database show that an improvement in median survival from seven to only 8.9 months has been obtained from 1972 to 1994 [49]. Although this is a disappointing acknowledgement, we will discuss some trials, which suggest that the situation has improved somewhat, since those early data were published.

Chemotherapy Standard for SCLC

For the most part, the combination of platinum (cisplatin or carboplatin) and etoposide are the chemotherapy standard of care. Complete response rates above 40% (with overall response rates above 80%) and median survival times of up to 14 months are reported with cisplatin and etoposide [50−52]. However, as stressed by Sundstrom and colleagues, most patients will relapse and die of their disease. Nevertheless, SCLC is potentially curable, since 3−8% of patients are long-term survivors [53−55]. Whereas, the five year survival for LS-SCLC is 7−15%, long-term survival is uncommon in extensive stage disease [56, 57].

When disease progresses, patients who remain well may be offered second-line chemotherapy with combinations such as CAV (cyclphosphamide, adriamycin and vincristine) or topotecan, although response rates to second-line chemotherapy are low (of the order of 20%) and survival is generally short [58, 59]. Therefore, although SCLC is a potentially chemosensitive disease, the vast majority of patients succumb within two years of diagnosis with the worldwide standard of care. Thus, much research has focused on trying to improve survival using different approaches which include the use of alternating drug regimens, dose-intensified chemotherapy, different cytotoxic agents and the use of novel biological agents.

Alternating Drug Regimens

In many centres etoposide and cisplatin remain the standard first-line treatment for limited disease although combinations such as CAV have proved activity as second-line treatment [58, 59]. These two drug regimens employ different modes of action, so alternating the regimens may maximize response by circumventing resistance. However, because studies investigating alternating regimens have provided contradictory results and failed to show a significant advantage, this approach has not been widely adopted [60, 61].

Dose-intensification of Chemotherapy for SCLC

A means by which to improve the results with combination chemotherapy in patients with SCLC is to increase the dose density of drug administration. Such approaches inevitably increase the potentially life-threatening haematological toxicity of treatment. Therefore prophylactic antibiotics, growth factor support and peripheral blood stem cell transplants have all been used to enable dose-intensification [62, 63]. Such approaches have demonstrated improved response rates and median survival in phase II studies. However, excess treatment-related fatalities are reported and several phase III trials have not shown a significant advantage over conventional dose therapy [64, 65]. One of the reasons given for the failure of these regimens to improve survival had been thought to be because it was difficult to deliver the desired dose intensity. Desired dose intensity was, however, achieved with one highly imaginative phase III study on better prognosis SCLC patients, which took the 4-weekly ICE (ifosfamide, carboplatin and etoposide) regimen, and delivered the chemotherapy 2-weekly with the aid of growth factors, supported by whole-blood haematopoietic progenitors after each cycle of chemotherapy. [66] This approach led to shorter treatment duration and less neutropenic sepsis than did standard ICE, but did not improve overall survival. There was also a considerable amount of work done more than a decade ago exploring the possible benefits of autologous bone marrow transplantation which equally failed to demonstrate a sufficient advantage to using this approach. Therefore in the UK at least, dose intensification is not regarded as a standard treatment (NICE document).

Novel Cytotoxic Agents and Combinations

In the last five years several new agents have been investigated in patients with SCLC. A number of phase II studies have reported encouraging response rates and survival with the agents such as paclitaxel, docetaxel and gemcitabine [67–71]. Randomized phase III data are awaited in order to ascertain whether these agents will offer any significant advantage over etoposide and platinum alone. A combination of particular interest is that of the topoisomerase I inhibitor irinotecan with cisplatin. In one phase II study this combination yielded a complete response rate of 29% and an overall response rate of 86% (median survival 13 months) in patients with ES-SCLC [72]. In a subsequent randomized phase III study an Irinotecan and Cisplatin combination was compared with etoposide and cisplatin in 154 patients with ES-SCLC [73]. The median survival (12.8 months) was significantly greater in the experimental arm than with the standard treatment (9.4 months). The combination of irinotecan and cisplatin was associated with less life-threatening myelosuppression, but more life-threatening diarrhoea than with the etoposide and cisplatin combination. However, in an earlier report of a 331 randomized patients, a modified weekly irinotecan and cisplatin regimen did not demonstrate a significant survival benefit over etoposide and cisplatin [74]. Thus, the role of irinotecan in the treatment of SCLC remains unclear at present.

The British Medical Research Council multicentre randomized LU21 trial looked at the novel combination of ICE-V (ifosfamide, carboplatin and etoposide with midcycle vincristine) versus standard chemotherapy in patients with good performance status SCLC [75]. Compared with standard chemotherapy, the ICE-V regimen improved overall survival (median survival = 15.6 months with ICE-V versus 11.6 months in controls) without quality-of-life penalties, despite an increased but manageable level of toxicity. Clearly, the novel ICE-V regimen holds promise and may be accepted as a new standard of care in the treatment of SCLC.

As for NSCLC the hope is that the new generation of targeted agents may also prove to have activity in SCLC. However to date phase I/II studies investigating EGFR and c-kit tyrosine kinase inhibitors, farnesyl transferase inhibitors, matrix metalloproteinase inhibitors, mTOR antagonists and vaccine therapy have been universally disappointing. Importantly Bevacizumab and other anti-angiogenic agents continue to be investigated and, we the authors feel, as discussed above by Thatcher *et al* in their paper on the MRC LU21 trial, that "the future probably lies with biologically targeted agents; SCLC exhibits numerous molecular abnormalities, including neuropeptide, gastrin-releasing peptide, CD117, and vascular endothelial growth factor expression, which may be exploitable" [75, 76]. Hopefully one of these approaches will yield positive results in the near future.

Conclusion

Chemotherapy for SCLC produces high response rates (up to 80%) and significantly prolongs survival (up to 30% two year survival for LS good performance patients – compared to just several weeks or months if no chemotherapy is given). However, these results are not hugely improved compared to two decades ago. It is proving difficult to improve further on the high response rates already observed, thus indicating that aiming to improve response rates further may not necessarily be the way to prolong survival. The lack of progress is in spite of much imaginative work with different combinations of drugs and different scheduling. Immensely imaginative work with dose intensity has also been of equitable disappointment. Studies using the new generation of targeted agents have so far proved disappointing in SCLC, but with improved understanding of the molecular mechanisms underlying these diseases, hopefully advances will be made in the near future. Novel systemic treatments (biological or chemotherapy) have translated into better results with other tumour types (some discussed above with respect to NSCLC), and we, the authors, agree with sentiments expressed in a recent publication (as discussed and referenced above) that the future lies with exploiting interventions with the numerous biological abnormalities exhibited by SCLC cells. It must of course be remembered that even though progress has been frustratingly slow in advancing survival for patients with SCLC, of this is a disease that most patients still derive enormous benefit from treatment with conventional chemotherapy. The benefits seen with the conventional ICE-V regimen discussed above could justify this becoming a new standard of care for the treatment of SCLC.

Historically, NSCLC has been regarded as relatively insensitive to chemotherapy but over the past decade, we have witnessed a revolution in the systemic treatment of this disease. Platinum doublets demonstrate improved survival and quality of life over best supportive care in the treatment of advanced-stage disease, and third generation platinum doublets (Taxol, Taxotere, Gemcitabine and Vinorelbine, with Cisplatin or Carboplatin) are associated with further improvements still. All these new drugs have given us an 'embarrassment of riches' though with no clear favourite regimen. There is not a treatment of choice for the first line treatment of advanced-stage disease, but rather a choice of treatments which should be on opted for the basis of familiarity with the chemotherapeutic regimen, expected toxicity, convenience of administration and costs. The exact role of cisplatin or carboplatin remains controversial, but the UK NCRI BTOG-2 study may answer this question. The role of novel biological agents in combination with first-line treatment is evolving. Small molecule tyrosine kinase inhibitors have so far provided disappointing results in this setting. However, results using antiangiogenic combination treatment with the endothelial growth factor (VEGF) antibody,

Bevacizumab, show promise. This could become a standard of care. Results from similar combination cytotoxic treatment and oral thalidomide (another antiangiogenic agent) are awaited from the results of a large UK NCRI study, which has just completed. There is also improved survival and quality of life with second line treatment, in the form of the cytotoxic drugs taxotere or pemetrexed, or the small molecule oral tyrosine kinase inhibitor, erlotinib. Erlotinib also improves quality of life and survival in the third treatment of advanced disease, provided both previous lines of treatment have been with cytotoxic drugs (i.e. a tyrosine kinase inhibitor has not already been used). In early-stage NSCLC, adjuvant chemotherapy (i.e. post-operative chemotherapy) has now become a standard of care, with either of the two third generation combinations, vinorelbine and cisplatin, or taxol and carboplatin, demonstrating the most significant survival advantages. The promising results seen with adjuvant UFT plus or minus cisplatin in Japan have not prompted Western World countries to use this regimen yet. There remains concern that that there might be a different pharacodynamic effect of drugs between Eastern and Western populations.

REFERENCES

1. Non Small Cell Lung Cancer Collaborative Group. (1995). Chemotherapy in non-small cell lung cancer: a meta-analysis using updated data on individual patients from 52 randomised clinical trials. *BMJ*, **311**, 899−909.
2. Cullen, M. H., Billingham, L. J., Woodroffe, C. M., *et al.* (1999). Mitomycin, ifosfamide, and cisplatin in unresectable non small cell lung cancer: effects on survival and quality of life, *J Clin Oncol*, **17**, 3188−94.
3. The Elderly Lung Cancer Vinorelbine Italian Study Group. (1999). Effects of vinorelbine on quality of life and survival of elderly patients with advanced non-small cell lung cancer. *J Natl Cancer Inst*, **91**, 66−72.
4. Ellis, P. A., Smith, I. E., Hardy, J. R., *et al.* (1995). Symptom relief with MVP (mitomycin C, vinblastine and cisplatin) chemotherapy in advanced non-small cell lung cancer, *Br J Cancer*, **71**, 366−70.
5. Depierre, A., Chastang, C., Quoix, E., *et al.* (1994). Vinorelbine versus vinorelbine plus cisplatin in advanced non small cell lung cancer: a randomised trial. *Ann Oncol*, **5**, 37−42.
6. Le Chevalier, T., Brisgand, D., Douillard, J. Y., *et al.* (1994). Randomised study of vinorelbine and cisplatin versus vindesine and cisplatin versus vinorelbine alone in advanced non small cell lung cancer: results of a European multicentre trial including 612 patients. *J Clin Oncol*, **12**, 360−7.

7. Wozniak, A. J., Crowley, J. J., Balcerzak, S. P., *et al.* (1998). Randomised trial comparing cisplatin with cisplatin plus vinorelbine in the treatment of advanced non small cell lung cancer: a Southwest Oncology Group Study. *J Clin Oncol*, **16**, 2459–65.

8. Cardenal, F., Lopez-Cabrerizo, M. P., Anton, A., *et al.* (1999). Randomised phase III study of gemcitabine-cisplatin versus etoposide-cisplatin in the treatment of locally advanced or metastatic non small cell lung cancer. *J Clin Oncol*, **17**, 12–18.

9. Crino, L., Scagliotti, G. V., Ricci, S., *et al.* (1999). Gemcitabine and cisplatin versus mitomycin, ifosfamide, and cisplatin in advanced non-small cell lung cancer: a randomised phase III study of the Italian Lung Cancer Project. *J Clin Oncol*, **17**, 3522–30.

10. Sandler, A. B., Nemunaitis, J., Denham, C., *et al.* (2000). Phase III trial of gemcitabine plus cisplatin versus cisplatin alone in patients with locally advanced or metastatic non small cell lung cancer. *J Clin Oncol*, **18**, 122–30.

11. Giaccone, G., Splinter, T. A., Debruyne, C., *et al.* (1998). Randomised study of paclitaxel-cisplatin versus cisplatin-teniposide in patients with advanced non small cell lung cancer. The European Organisation for the Research and Treatment of Cancer Lung Cancer Cooperative Group. *J Clin Oncol*, **16**, 2133–41.

12. Bonomi, P., Kim, K., Fairclough, D., *et al.* (2000). Comparison of survival and quality of life in advanced non small cell lung cancer patients treated with two dose levels of paclitaxel combined with cisplatin versus etoposide with cisplatin: results of an Eastern Cooperative Oncology Group trial. *J Clin Oncol*, **18**, 623–31.

13. Schiller, J. H., Harrington, D., Belani, C. P., *et al.* (2002). Comparison of four chemotherapy regimens for advanced non small cell lung cancer. *N Engl J Med*, **346**, 92–8.

14. The diagnosis and treatment of lung cancer. National Collaborating Centre for Acute Care, Commissioned by National Institute of Clinical Excellence document, February 2005.

15. Rodriquez, J., Parvel, J., Pluzanska, A., *et al.* (2001). A multicenter randomized phase III study of docetaxel and carboplatin versus vinorelbine and cisplatin in chemotherapy-naive patients with advanced and metastatic non-small cell lung cancer. *Proceedings of the American Society of Clinical Oncology*, abstract 314.

16. Ettinger, D. S. (2002). Is there a preferred combination chemotherapy regimen for metastatic non small cell lung cancer? The *Oncologist*, **7**, 226–33.

17. Le Chevalier, T., Scagliotti, G., Natale, R., *et al.* (2005). Efficacy of gemcitabine plus platinum chemotherapy compared with other platinum-containing regimens in advanced non-small cell lung cancer: a meta-analysis of survival outcomes. *Lung Cancer*, **47**, 69–80.

18. Cornella, P., Frasci, G., Panza, N., *et al.* (2000). Randomised trial comparing cisplatin, gemcitabine, and vinorelbine with either cisplatin and gemcitabine or cisplatin and vinorelbine in advanced non-small cell lung cancer: interim analysis of a phase III trial of the Southern Italy Cooperative Oncology Group. *J Clin Oncol*, **18**, 1451–7.

19. Georgoulias, V., Ardavanis, A., Tsiafaki, X., *et al.* (2005). Vinorelbine plus cisplatin versus docetaxel plus gemcitabine in advanced non-small cell lung cancer: a phase III randomised trial, *J Clin Oncol*, **23**, 2937–45.

20. Hotta, K., Matsuo, K., Ueoka, H., *et al.* (2004). Meta-analysis of randomized clinical trials comparing cisplatin to carboplatin in patients with advanced non-small cell lung cancer, *J Clin Oncol*, **22**, 3852–59.

21. Roszkowski, K., Pluzanska, A., Krzakowski, M., *et al.* (2000). A multicentre, randomized, phase III study of docetaxel plus best supportive care versus best supportive care in chemotherapy-naïve patients with metastatic or non-resectable localized non-small cell lung cancer. *Lung Cancer*, **27**, 145–57.

22. Shepherd, F. A., Dancey, J., Ramlau, R., *et al.* (2000). Prospective randomized trial of docetaxel versus best supportive care in patients with non-small cell lung cancer previously treated with platinum-based chemotherapy. *J Clin Oncol*, **18**, 2095–103.

23. Hanna, N., Shepherd, F. A., Fossella, F. V., *et al.* (2004). Randomized phase III trial of pemetrexed versus docetaxel in patients with non-small cell lung cancer previously treated with chemotherapy. *J Clin Oncol*, **22**, 1589–97.

24. Mountain, C. (1997). Revisions in the International System for Staging Lung Cancer. *Chest*, **111**, 1710–17.

25. Arriagada, R., Bergman, B., Dunant, A., *et al.* (2004). Cisplatin-based adjuvant chemotherapy in patients with completely resected non-small cell lung cancer. *N Engl J Med*, **350**, 351–60.

26. Strauss, G. M., Herndon, J., Maddaus, M. A., *et al.* (2004). Randomised clinical trial of adjuvant chemotherapy with paclitaxel and carboplatin following resection in stage IB non-small cell lung cancer: report of Cancer and Leukaemia Group B (CALGB) protocol 9633. *Proceedings of American Society of Clinical Oncology*, abstract 621.

27. Winton, T., Livingston, R., Johnson, D., *et al.* (2005). Vinorelbine plus cisplatin versus observation in resected non-small cell lung cancer. *N Engl J Med*, **352**, 2589–97.

28. Douillard, J., Rosell, R., Delena, M., *et al.* (2005). ANITA: Phase III adjuvant vinorelbine and cisplatin versus observation in completely resected (stage I-III) non-small cell lung cancer patients:final results after 70 month median follow-up. On behalf of Adjuvant Navelbine International Trialist Association. *Proceedings of the American Society of Clinical Oncology*, abstract 7013.

29. Scagliotti, G. V., Foassati, R., Torri, V., *et al.* (2003). Randomised study of adjuvant chemotherapy for completely resected stage I, II or IIIA non-small cell lung cancer. *J Natl Cancer Inst*, **95**, 1453–61.

30. Keller, S. M., Adak, S., Wagner, H., *et al.* (2000). A randomized trial of postoperative adjuvant treatment in patients with completely resected stage II or IIIa non-small cell lung cancer. *N Engl J Med*, **343**, 1217–22.

31. Waller, D., Peake, M. D., Stephens, R. J., *et al.* (2004). Chemotherapy for patients with non-small cell lung cancer: the surgical setting of the Big Lung Trial. *Eur J cardiothoracic Surg*, **26**, 173–82.

32. Visbal, A. L., Leighl, N. B., Feld, R., Shepherd, F. A. (2005). Adjuvant chemotherapy for early-stage non-small cell lung cancer. *Chest*, **128**, 2933—43.

33. Hotta, K., Matsuo, K., Ueoka, H., *et al.* (2004). Role of adjuvant chemotherapy in patients with resected non-small cell lung cancer: reappraisal with a meta-analysis of randomized controlled trials. *J Clin Oncol*, **22**, 3860—7.

34. Comets, E., Ikeda, K., Hoff, P., *et al.* (2003). Comparison of the pharmacokinetics of S-1, an oral anti-cancer agent in Western and Japanese patients. *J Pharmacokinetic and Pharmacodyn*, **30**, 257—83.

35. Depierre, A., Milleron, B., Moro-Sibilot, D., *et al.* (2002). Preoperative chemotherapy followed by surgery compared with primary surgery in respectable stage I (except T1N0), II and IIIa non-small cell lung cancer. *J Clin Oncol*, **20**, 247—53.

36. Pisters, K., Vallieres, E., Bunn, P., *et al.* (2005). S9900: A phase III trial of surgery alone or surgery plus preoperative paclitaxel/carboplatin chemotherapy in early-stage non-small cell lung cancer: preliminary results. *Proceedings of the American Society of Clinical Oncology*, abstract 7012.

37. Rosell, R., Cobo, M., Isla, D., *et al.* (2005). ERCC mRNA-based randomized phase III trial of docetaxel doublets with cisplatin or gemcitabine in stage IV non-small cell lung cancer patients. *Proceedings of the American Society of Clinical Oncology*, abstract 7002.

38. Fukuoka, M., Yano, S., Giaccone, G., *et al.* (2003). Multi-institutional randomized phase II trial of gefitinib for previously treated patients with advanced non-small cell lung cancer. *J Clin Oncol*, **21**, 2237—46.

39. Kris, M. G., Natale, R. B., Herbst, R. S., *et al.* (2002). A phase II trial of ZD 1839 (Iressa) in advanced non-small cell lung cancer patients who had failed platinum- and docetaxel-based regimens (IDEAL 2). *Proceedings of the American Society of Clinical Oncology*, abstract 292.

40. Giaccone, G., Herbst, R. S., Manegold, C., *et al.* (2004). Gefitinib in combination with gemcitabine and cisplatin in advanced non-small cell lung cancer: a phase III trial: INTACT 1. *J Clin Oncol*, **22**, 777—84.

41. Herbst, R. S., Prager, D., Hermann, R., *et al.* (2004). TRIBUTE-a phase III trial of erlotinib (OSI-774) combined with carboplatin and paclitaxel chemotherapy in advanced non-small cell lung cancer. *Proceedings of the Amercian Society of Clinical Oncology*, abstract 7011.

42. Gatzemeier, U., Pluzanska, A., Szczesna, A., *et al.* Results of a phase III trial of erlotinib (OSI-774) combined with cisplatin and gemcitabine chemotherapy in advanced non-small cell lung cancer. *Proceedings of the American Society of Clinical Oncology*, abstract 7010.

43. Shepherd, F. A., Pereira, J., Ciuleanu, T. E., *et al.* (2004). A randomized placebo-controlled trial of erlotinib in patients with advanced non-small cell lung cancer following failure of 1st line or 2nd line chemotherapy, A National Cancer Institute of Canada Clinical Trials Group Trial. *Proceedings of the American Society of Oncology*, abstract 7022.

44. Lynch, T. J., Bell, D. W., Sordella, R., *et al.* (2004). Activating mutations in the epidermal growth factor receptor underlying responsiveness of non-small cell lung cancer to gefitinib. *N Engl J Med*, **350**, 2129—39.

45. Sandler, A. B., Gray, R., Brahmer, J., *et al.* Randomized phase II/III trial of paclitaxel/carboplatin with or without bevacizumab in patients with advanced non-squamous non-small cell lung cancer: an Eastern Cooperative Oncology Group study: E4599. *Proceedings of the American Society of Oncology*, abstract 4.

46. Fanucchi, M. P., Fossella, F., Fidias, P., *et al.* (2005). Bortezomib +/− docetaxel in previously treated patients with advanced non-small cell lung cancer: a phase II study. *Proceedings of the American Society of Clinical Oncology*, abstract 7034.

47. Lynch, T. J., Lilenbaum, R., Bonomi, P., *et al.* (2004). A phase II trial of cetuximab as therapy for recurrent non-small cell lung cancer. *Proceedings of the American Society of Clinical Oncology*, abstract 7084.

48. Johnson, B. E. and Heymach, J. V. (2004). Farnesyl transferase inhibitors for patients with lung cancer. *Clinical Cancer Research*, **10**, 4254s−5457s.

49. Chute, J. P., Chen, T., Feigel, E., *et al.* (1999). Twenty years of phase III trials for patients with extensive-stage small cell lung cancer: perceptible progress. *J Clin Oncol*, **17**, 1794−1801.

50. Evans, W. K., Osoba, D., Shepherd, F. A., *et al.* (1985). Etoposide (VP-16) and cisplatin: an effective treatment for relapse in small-cell lung. *J Clin Oncol*, **3**, 65−71.

51. Einhorn, L. H., Crawford, J., Birch, R., *et al.* (1988). Cisplatin plus etoposide consolidation following cyclophosphamide, doxorubicin, and vincristine in limited small-cell lung cancer. *J Clin Oncol*, **6**, 451−6.

52. Sundstrom, S., Bremnes, R. M., Kaasa, S., *et al.* (2002). Cisplatin and etoposide regimen is superior to cyclophosphamide, epirubicin, and Vincristine regimen in small-cell lung cancer: results from a randomised phase III trial with 5 years' follow-up. *J Clin Oncol*, **20**, 4665−72.

53. Souhami, R. L., Law, K. (1990). *Longevity in small cell lung cancer: A report to the Lung Cancer Subcommittee of the United Kingdom Coordinating Committee for Cancer Research*, **61**, 584−9.

54. Lassen, U., Osterlind, K., Hansen, M., *et al.* (1995). Long-term survival in small-cell lung cancer: post treatment characteristics in patients surviving 5 to 18+ years: an analysis of 1,714 consecutive patients. *J Clin Oncol* **13**, 1215−20.

55. Watkin, S. W., Hayhurst, G. K., Green, J. A. (1990). Time trends in the outcome of lung cancer management: A study of 9090 cases diagnosed in the Mersey Region, 1974−86. *Br J Cancer*, **61**, 590−6.

56. Sandler, A. B. (1997). Current management of small cell lung cancer. *Semin Oncol*, **24**, 463−76.

57. Kelly, K. (2000). New chemotherapy agents for small cell lung cancer. *Chest*, **111**(Suppl 1), 156S−162S.

58. von Pawel, J., Schiller, Shepherd, *et al.* (1999). Topotecan Versus Cyclophosphamide, Doxorubicin, and Vincristine for the Treatment of Recurrent Small-Cell Lung Cancer. *J Clin Oncol*, **17**, 658−67.

59. Huisman, C., Postmus, P. E., Giaccone, G., Smit, E. F. (1999). Second-line chemotherapy and its evaluation in small-cell lung cancer. *Cancer Treat Rev*, **25**, 199−206.

60. Roth, B. J., Johnson, D. H., Einhorn, L. H., *et al.* (1992). Randomized study of cyclophosphamide, doxorubicin, and vincristine versus etoposide and cisplatin versus alternation of these two regimens in extensive small-cell lung cancer: A phase III trial of the Southeastern Cancer Study Group. *J Clin Oncol*, **10**, 282–91.

61. Fukuoka, M., Furuse, K., Saijo, N., *et al.* (1991). Randomized trial of cyclophosphamide, doxorubicin and vincristine versus cisplatin and etoposide versus alteration of these regimens in small-cell lung cancer. *J Natl Cancer Inst*, **83**, 855–61.

62. Tjan-Heijen, V. C., Postmus, P. E., Ardizzoni, A., *et al.* (2001). Reduction of chemotherapy-induced febrile leucopenia by prophylactic use of ciprofloxacin and roxithromycin in small-cell lung cancer patients: an EORTC double-blind placebo-controlled phase III study. *Ann Oncol*, **12**, 1359–68.

63. Steward, W. P., Von Pawel, J., Gatzemeier, U., *et al.* (1998). Effects of granulocyte-macrophage colony-stimulating factor and dose-intensification of V-ICE chemotherapy in small cell lung cancer: a prospective randomized study of 300 patients. *J Clin Oncol*, **16**, 642–50.

64. Murray, N., Livingston, R. B., Shepherd, F. A., *et al.* (1999). Randomised study of CODE versus alternating CAV/EP for extensive-stage small cell lung cancer: an intergroup study of the National Cancer Institute of Canada Clinical Trials Group and the Southwest Oncology Group. *J Clin Oncol*, **17**, 2300–8.

65. Furuse, K., Fukuoka, M., Nishiwaki, Y., *et al.* (1998). Phase III study of intensive weekly chemotherapy with recombinant granulocyte colony-stimulating factor versus standard chemotherapy in extensive disease small-cell lung cancer. *J Clin Oncol*, **16**, 2126–32.

66. Lorigan, P., Woll, P. J., O'Brien, *et al.* (2005). randomized phase III trial of dose-dense chemotherapy supported by whole-blood hematopoietic progenitors in better-prognosis small-cell lung cancer. *J Natl Cancer Inst*, **97**, 666–74. Erratum in: *J Natl Cancer Inst*, 97, 941.

67. Kelly, K., pan, Z., Wood, M. E., *et al.* (1999). A phase I study of paclitaxel, etoposide and cisplatin in extensive-stage small cell lung cancer. *Clin Cancer Res*, **5**, 3419–24.

68. Glisson, B. S., Kurie, J. M., Perez-Soler, R., *et al.* (1999). Cisplatin, etoposide, and paclitaxel in the treatment of patients with extensive samll cell lung cancer. *J Clin Oncol*, **17**, 2309–15.

69. Earle, C. C., Stewart, D. J., Cormier, Y., *et al.* (1998). A phase I study of gemcitabine/cisplatin/etoposide in the treatment of small-cell lung cancer. *Lung Cancer*, **22**, 235–41.

70. Hesketh, P. J., Crowley, J. J., Burris, III H. A., *et al.* (1999). Evaluation of docetaxel in previously untreated extensive-stage small cell lung cancer: a Southwest Oncology Group Trial. *Cancer J Sci Am*, **5**, 237–41.

71. Kirschling, R. J., Grill, J. P., Marks, R. S., *et al.* (1999). Paclitaxel and G-CSF in previously untreated patients with extensive stage small cell lung cancer: a phase II study of the North Central Cancer Treatment Group. *Am J Clin Oncol*, **22**, 517–22.

72. Kudoh, S., Fujiwara, Y., Takada, H., *et al.* (1998). Phase II study of irinotecan combined with cisplatin in patients with previously untreated small-cell lung cancer. West Japan Lung Cancer Group. *J Clin Oncol*, **16**, 1068–74.

73. Noda, K., Nishiwaki, Y., Kawahara, M., *et al.* (2002). Irinotecan plus cisplatin compared with etoposide plus cisplatin for extensive small cell lung cancer. *N Engl J Med*, **346**, 85–91.

74. Hanna, N. H., Einhorn, L., Sandler, A., *et al.* (2005). Randomized, phase III trial comparing irinotecan/cisplatin (IP) with etoposide/cisplatin (EP) in patients (pts) with previously untreated, extensive stage (ES) small cell lung cancer (SCLC). *J Clin Oncol*, **23**, 1094 (suppl; abstr 7004).

75. Thatcher, N., Qian, W., Clark, *et al.* (2005). Ifosfamide, Carboplatin and Etoposide With Midcycle Vincristine Versus Standard Chemotherapy in Patients With Small-Cell Lung Cancer and Good Performance Status: Clinical and Quality-of-life Results of the British Medical Research Council Multicenter Randomised LU21 Trial. *J Clin Oncol*, **23**, 8371–9.

76. Wakelee, H., Kelly, K. (2004). Novel approaches for the treatment of small-cell lung cancer. *Haematol Oncol Clin North Am*, **18**, 499–518.

8

Radiotherapy in Lung Cancer

Shahreen Ahmad

Department of Clinical Oncology, St Thomas' Hospital, London, UK

Introduction

Lung cancer is the second most common malignancy diagnosed in men after prostate cancer and third most common after breast and colorectal in women. In 2000, there were 38,410 new cases of lung cancer diagnosed in the UK [1]. Incidence increases with age, with the most prevalent age group being the over 75s. As indicated in the chapter on chemotherapy for non-small cell lung cancer (NSCLC), survival rates remain low for patients treated with chemotherapy alone. Radiotherapy is an alternative modality of treatment which offers improved survival advantage to those with locally advanced disease.

Small cell lung cancer is a chemosensitive tumour. Nevertheless, studies have shown that radiotherapy can improve local control in patients who achieve a complete response following chemotherapy and who have disease localized to the chest [2]. There are also data that suggest that some of these patients benefit from prophylactic cranial irradiation, in the absence of proven brain metastases [3].

A further important role for radiotherapy in lung cancer patients is to treat symptomatic metastatic disease. This is usually in the palliative setting and the location of the metastatic deposit has a bearing on whether radiotherapy is suitable or not. However, radiation therapy can be an extremely effective treatment for symptoms such as pain, haemoptysis and cough [4, 5]. There are certain situations where emergency or urgent radiotherapy is the treatment of choice (e.g. spinal cord compression). Patients are treated in a multidisciplinary setting to ensure optimum management of each individual case. Particularly important in the palliative setting is the patient's general condition and factors affecting quality of life. These issues are assessed in the performance status for each patient which is based on level of daily activity and general well-being. It is a useful tool in deciding the most appropriate treatment for the lung cancer patient.

Non-small Cell Lung Cancer (NSCLC)

Radical Radiotherapy for NSCLC

The majority of patients who receive radical radiotherapy as their definitive treatment for NSCLC are those with locally advanced disease. These are patients whose disease is limited to the thorax but is too extensive for surgical resection and usually have bulky Stage IIIA or IIIB lesions. These patients will usually receive combination treatment with platinum-based chemotherapy and radical radiotherapy, usually a fractionated course to a total dose in the region of 64 Gray in 32 fractions.

A proportion of patients with Stage I and II disease will be unsuitable for surgery due to poor lung function or other medical problems and these patients are often suitable for treatment with radical radiotherapy. If the volume to be irradiated is small, the radiation may be hypofractionated to reduce the overall treatment time, treating with 55 Gray in four weeks. If the volume is large, a similar regime to that used for locally advanced Stage III disease can be implemented.

There are a number of side effects of radical radiation treatment including skin toxicity, fatigue and rib pain. The important side effects which determine the maximum dose of radiation delivered to a patient are called dose-limiting side effects and the normal tissues affected are termed organs at risk (OAR). For lung radiation the dose-limiting side effects are pneumonitis and oesophagitis with the spinal cord being an additional OAR.

Early radiation damage in pneumonitis is characterized by injury to the small vessels and capillaries with the formation of vascular congestion and increased vascular permeability. At this stage a fibrin-rich exudate is present in the alveolar spaces. Following on from this, there is obstruction of pulmonary capillaries by platelets, fibrin and collagen. Type II pneumocytes become hyperplastic and the alveolar walls can become infiltrated with fibroblasts. In the fibrosis phase, the histopathological characteristics that dominate are vascular subintimal fibrosis, thickening of the alveolar walls and luminal narrowing.

Certain factors are critical to the development of radiation pneumonitis. The most important factor is the volume of lung irradiated. The total dose of radiation and the fractionation schedule also contribute to the extent of pneumonitis. Other factors to consider are smoking history, increasing age of the patient and pre-existing lung disease, as well as concurrent drug therapy especially in the form of chemotherapy. The PORT meta-analysis (examining the effect of post-operative radiotherapy in NSCLC) reported a worse overall survival for patients who received radiotherapy following surgery compared to those who received surgery alone [11, 12] The non-cancer related deaths that occurred in these patients were due mainly to fatal pneumonitis. Numerous studies recently have addressed the issue of radiotherapy dose escalation for NSCLC and also various combinations of chemotherapy with radiotherapy schedules. These provide invaluable data on response and survival as well as detailed information on toxicity associated with radiation.

A number of Phase III randomized trials [6, 13] have reported improved response rates of concurrent chemoradiotherapy over sequential treatment at the expense of increased toxicity. One of the main toxicities encountered with concurrent therapy is acute oesophagitis. Groups have reported models to predict the development of radiation-induced oesophagitis [14, 15]. The consensus opinion is that whereas some parameters, such as mean oesophageal dose, maximal oesophageal dose and the addition of concurrent chemotherapy have an effect on outcome; other parameters such as length or volume of oesophagus irradiated may not be as important as previously assumed. [16]

Numerous groups are currently examining how far it is possible to dose escalate radiation in NSCLC patients who are treated radically and this is largely dependent on normal tissue tolerance, especially oesophagus and lung tissue.

Adjuvant Radiotherapy in NSCLC

An integral part of the management of a number of tumour types such as breast cancer and rectal cancer is local radiotherapy given post-operatively as an adjuvant treatment to reduce the risk of local recurrence. The role of adjuvant radiotherapy in lung cancer is less clear. In cases where there has been an incomplete resection at surgery or a pathologically proven metastases has been found in the mediastinal nodes, local radiotherapy to the areas at risk may be beneficial. The PORT meta-analysis [11, 12] showed that giving radiotherapy in N0/1 patients was detrimental and therefore is not offered to these patients. However, the PORT meta-analysis is based on old trials with older radiotherapy techniques which are not used today. Current trials with modern radiation techniques are in development stages and will be recruiting soon.

There are occasions during the surgical treatment of non-small cell lung cancer when it is not possible to achieve clear resection margins. This is often due to the fact that disease is present closer to major organs such as pulmonary trunk or cardiac tissue than was initially envisaged on pre-operative imaging. In these cases, incomplete resection margins may occur macroscopically or microscopically. These patients will normally be offered post-operative adjuvant radiotherapy. There are no randomized data addressing the benefit of radiotherapy in this situation, but a number of comparative non-randomized studies have indicated that the recurrence rate is higher if radiotherapy is not given [21, 22].

Radiotherapy Fractionation and Delivery

Animal models have demonstrated that rapid repopulation occurs in lung cancer cells, especially squamous cell subtype [17, 18]. A way of exploiting this fact radiobiologically is to increase the number of radiation treatments given in a 24 hour period. This is known as hyperfractionation. Radiation delivery can also be *accelerated* by reducing the overall treatment time for a course of treatment. Tumour cell proliferation during the treatment reduces the efficacy of radiotherapy and reducing the overall treatment time reduces the rate of repopulation of tumour cells. Saunders *et al* devised the CHART regime (continuous hyperfractionated accelerated radiotherapy) where patients were treated with three 1.5 Gy fractions of radiotherapy/day for 12 consecutive days to a total dose of 54 Gy. This was compared to the conventional radiation schedule for lung cancer at the time (60 Gy in 30 fractions over six weeks). Significant benefits in incidence of local recurrence as well as survival were seen for CHART patients. A total of 563 patients with non-small cell lung cancer and Head and Neck cancer were entered between 1990 and 1995. The survival probability for patients treated with CHART at two years was 30% compared to 21% in non-CHART patients. The improved effect of CHART was particularly significant for squamous cell cancers [19, 20]. However, significantly greater rates of toxicity were noted in the CHART patients including oesophagitis and lung pneumonitis and fibrosis. The CHART studies are now being repeated around the world and a current UK trial is underway investigating the additional benefit of chemotherapy with CHART — the INCH trial.

Other issues surrounding delivery of radiation include dose escalation. Increasing the dose of radiation increases the probability of tumour cell kill but also causes greater normal tissue toxicity. Balancing these two factors will achieve the optimum therapeutic ratio when treating the patient. Numerous groups are currently examining how far it is possible to dose escalate radiation in NSCLC patients who are treated radically, and this is largely dependent on normal tissue tolerance, especially oesophagus and lung tissue.

There is increasing evidence that the combination of chemotherapy and radio-therapy for NSCLC is superior to radiotherapy alone or chemotherapy alone, in terms of five-year and median survival for patients with locally advanced disease [6–9]. The high rate of distant metastases provided the rationale for adding chemotherapy to the established localized radiotherapy treatment. Following the acceptance of the combined approach to treatment, research has more recently been directed at investigating the optimum manner of delivery. The combination of chemotherapy with radiotherapy is doubly beneficial as chemotherapy has an independent effect on the tumour cells and can also act as a radiation sensitizer, causing the tumour cells to be more vulnerable to the cytotoxic effect of radiation. The question of whether the chemotherapy should be given sequentially or concur-rently with radiation remains somewhat controversial. Several randomized trials have directly compared concurrent with sequential treatment and suggest improved survival with the concomitant approach at the expense of increased toxicity. [8, 9, 10]. A current British trial is addressing this question currently (SOCCAR trial).

Small Cell Lung Cancer (SCLC)

Radiotherapy in Limited-stage SCLC

SCLC is, first and foremost, a chemosensitive disease. Nevertheless, up to 80% of patients treated with chemotherapy develop local recurrences. There is evidence (from two meta-analyses) that thoracic radiation in patients who have limited-stage disease improves survival (5% at 2 years) and doubles local control [23, 24]. The benefits of radiotherapy are greatest in patients who have achieved a complete response to chemotherapy and are of good performance status. The optimum dose for thoracic radiation in SCLC patients is controversial. Studies show that there is a major advantage in increasing the dose from 35 to 40 Gy; a further small benefit can be achieved up to 50 Gy but no real benefit in increasing the dose further [25, 26, 27]. Other controversial areas include whether to treat mediastinal nodes electively and the sequencing of chemotherapy and radiotherapy [28, 29].

Prophylactic Cranial Irradiation (PCI)

Up to 50% of long-term survivors with small cell lung cancer will develop brain metastases. In some patients, prophylactic irradiation of the whole brain can be

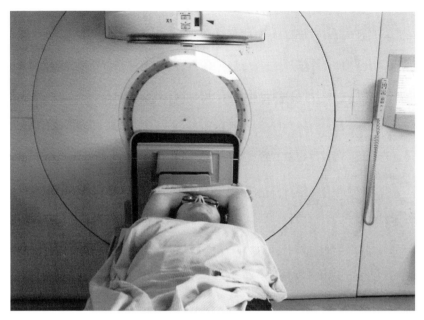

**Figure 8.1 Lung cancer patient in treatment position on linear accelerator couch for radiotherapy
(for a colour version of this figure please see the colour plate section)**

beneficial. A meta-analysis by Auperin *et al* in 1999 [3] showed that PCI yielded
a 5.6% three-year survival advantage in patients with limited-stage disease who
achieved a complete response to chemotherapy. Whole brain radiotherapy is therefore recommended to a dose of 25–30 Gy in 10 fractions for good performance
status patients who have a good response to chemotherapy.

Modern Radiotherapy Techniques

Megavoltage (MV) radiation which is used in the treatment of NSCLC is artificially
produced from a machine called a linear accelerator (linac). The energy of radiation
varies between 4 to 25 MV in most linacs. Patients lie supine on a couch with their
arms supported above their heads (Fig. 8.1) while radiation is emitted from the
head of the linac. Each treatment takes approximately 10 minutes to deliver and
the patient is free breathing during this time. Patients have permanent marks
or 'radiation tattoos' placed on their skin to minimize day-to-day set-up error.
The room housing the linear accelerator is also furnished with laser lights to line
up the tattoos for daily treatment. The patient's position for treatment must be

comfortable, reproducible and suitable for acquisitions of images for planning and treatment delivery.

Image Acquisition: Conventional versus CT Planning

Techniques for delivering radiation have improved dramatically over the last 10 years and continue to do so. Previously, radiotherapy treatment was planned using fluoroscopic visualization of the region of interest with a conventional radio-therapy simulator. This machine is still used for palliative treatments as well as for treatment verification purposes but is not in the radical treatment of lung cancer. The advent of 3-Dimensional (3D) conformal radiotherapy with CT planning has revolutionized radical radiotherapy and has enabled us to give high doses of radi-ation with acceptable normal tissue toxicity. The technique uses target volumes delineated on CT slices at multiple levels through the patient over the region of interest, on which normal structures are also outlined. A plan can then be constructed using multiple coplanar fields to treat the lung tumour according to the delineated target volume while calculating the dose of radiation to the normal tisuues (Fig. 8.2).

Treatment Verification

Geometric verification of anatomical regions of interest to measure day-to-day variation in set-up can be achieved in a number of ways. The most widely used methods at present are to acquire a radiograph taken on the treatment unit (portal film) or by real-time visualization of the patient using an online electronic portal imaging device (EPID). However, a major disadvantage of these methods is that the treatment machines emit megavoltage photons making the anatomical resolution of images very poor. Newer methods utilise Image Guided Radiotherapy tech-niques (IGRT), such as cone beam (CT) linear accelerators. On these treatment units, either a CT or fluoroscopic kilovoltage attachment is present on the treat-ment machine so that high quality images of the patient can be taken during treatment. IGRT takes into account differences between individual patients, has the ability to alter radiotherapy treatment plans during a course of treatment and therefore allows customization of treatment for the individual. 3D conformal

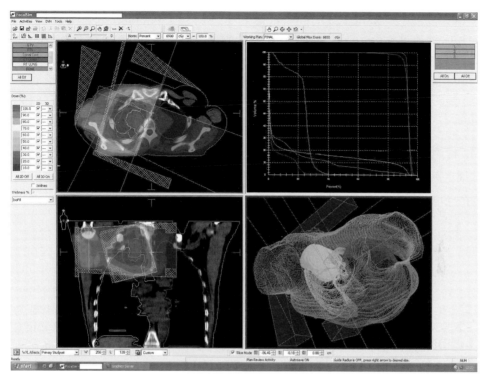

Figure 8.2 Radiotherapy treatment plan for lung tumour. Colour washes indicate percentage isodose to patient target volume (for a colour version of this figure please see the colour plate section)

radiotherapy planning systems are used in most Radiotherapy Centres in the UK at present, with many centres currently commissioning the newer equipment available to improve treatment delivery yet further.

Target Volume Definition

Target volume definition is an essential part of the radiotherapy planning process and obviously impacts on response and progression rates. It is important to define the target volume correctly and accurately allowing for tumour motion with respiration, and cover all involved disease as well as considering treatment of at-risk tissue and nodes.

CT scanning is the primary imaging modality used to define target volumes for radiation. Three target volume definitions are stipulated by the International

Commission on Radiation Units (ICRU) [30, 31] to aid in radiotherapy planning. These are gross tumour volume (GTV), which includes the macroscopic tumour as visible on examination of the patient and using imaging scans, the clinical target volume (CTV), which is the GTV with a margin added to account for microscopic spread of malignant cells around the tumour, and planning target volume (PTV), which constitutes the CTV with a margin added for internal organ motion and technical radiation set-up errors. The ICRU 62 report includes an additional volume between CTV and PTV, called the Internal Target Volume (ITV). The factors to consider when adding a margin from CTV to ITV are internal organ motion and then separately add a margin for set-up errors between ITV and PTV.

To try and account for these errors in a systematic and consistent way, many radiotherapy departments have specific protocols devised to guide the clinician in choosing appropriate target volumes. Typical margins that are used are 1 cm around the GTV with up to 1.5 cm in the cranio-caudal direction [34, 35].

Intensity Modulated Radiation Therapy (IMRT)

The relatively new technique of IMRT, intensity modulation within a radiation beam, is designed on the basis of the target prescription and a set of dose constraints for sensitive structures using inverse planning algorithms. The capability of differentiating the weight of individual rays of a beam in IMRT allows sculpting of the isodose distributions to achieve maximum dose conformity.

IMRT has been used with considerable success in certain tumour sites including head and neck and prostate cancer, and its role in NSCLC is emerging. The issues to consider are the motion of the tissues and inhomogeneity of the region, which may cause dose deviation and uncertainty, causing adverse effects on both tumours and normal tissue. A study by Grills *et al* 2003 [32] compared 3D conformal radiotherapy to IMRT plans in 18 patients with NSCLC whose disease ranged between Stages I to IIIB. In terms of lung and oesophagus toxicity, a benefit was seen in selected patients, namely those who were node positive or had tumours in close proximity to the oesophagus, with the IMRT plans compared to 3D conformal plans. However, the same advantage was not seen in node negative patients. This may be due to the fact that use of multiple beam angles and intensity modulation may increase the integral radiation dose delivered to the lungs, thus increasing the possibility of treatment-induced toxicity. Other studies have demonstrated significant advantages of IMRT over 3D conformal radiotherapy in non-small cell lung cancer [33].

Therefore, although it is known that 3D conformal radiotherapy is a safe and efficient technique for use in the radical treatment of NSCLC, the same cannot be said for IMRT. Further studies are required to evaluate the technique in lung cancer patients and work is needed to improve radiation delivery using IMRT.

Palliative Radiotherapy

Radiotherapy can also be useful in palliation of symptoms associated with lung cancer. Patients who have disease in the chest that is too extensive to treat with radical intent can gain considerable relief from their symptoms with palliative radiotherapy to the chest. Typical dose schedules include 39 Gy in 13 fractions, 17 Gy in two fractions and 10 Gy in a single fraction. The Medical Research Council Lung Cancer Working Party found a better symptomatic response as well as improved median survival for the higher dose schedule and therefore this is the treatment of choice in good performance patients. [43–46]. However, it should be noted that the majority of lung cancer patients with incurable disease who require palliation of symptoms are not candidates for fractionated high-dose radiotherapy schedules. For the majority, a poor performance status precludes higher dose treatment and one or two fractions of treatment provides adequate palliation of symptoms without significant side effects or impact on quality-of-life [47]. The features most likely to respond to palliative chest radiotherapy include haemoptysis, symptoms of superior vena caval obstruction, chest pain and cough. Radiotherapy can also be used to treat metastatic disease including painful bone metastases, brain metastases and spinal cord compression. Patients with a single solitary brain metastasis or a single level of spinal cord compression from a metastatic deposit may benefit from surgical intervention which offers the greatest opportunity for long-term control. These patients are normally otherwise fit and well and have no other sites of relapse from their disease. They will usually receive post-operative radiotherapy to further extend long-term control.

Endobronchial radiotherapy treatment using an intracavitary brachytherapy technique is sometimes used for patients with intrinsic compression from a tumour. There is no clear evidence of improved response or survival with this method over external beam radiotherapy, however it can be useful in specific circumstances where external beam treatment is not possible.

Future Developments

Use of Positron Emmision Tomography (PET) Scanning in Target Volume Definition and Radiotherapy Planning

PET (and PET/CT) scanning is a sensitive and specific imaging tool to identify lung tumours and mediastinal nodes. It is particularly useful at differentiating tumour mass from adjacent consolidated lung tissue or atelectasis. This could then enable radiotherapy treatment target volumes to be reduced and minimize irradiating uninvolved lung tissue. A number of planning studies have been carried out to assess the impact of PET on radiotherapy planning and a significant effect was seen on the volume. PET also accurately identifies thoracic nodes with tumour metastases and patterns of lymph node spread on lung cancer are currently being studied using PET in order to predict nodes at risk of metastases in ling cancer.

Movement of Lung Tumours with Respiration

The movement of structures with respiration has a significant impact on the size, shape and position of the PTV. Various methods have been employed recently to attempt to reduce the CTV to PTV margin in lung cancer. One technique is the utilization of gated radiotherapy [36, 37]. The basic concept of this technique is to gate the radiation beam in some way as the patient breathes freely. Short bursts of radiation can then be delivered repeatedly at a particular phase in the breathing cycle.

Another method is the Active Breathing Control (ABC) apparatus which aims to minimize the margin for breathing motion by stopping the breathing at specific points in the respiratory cycle. Wong *et al* 1999 [38] described the technique and their results in treating patients in this manner. The ABC apparatus consists of a modified ventilator with two separate flow monitors and two 'scissor valves' to monitor and control inspiration and expiration independently. The flow signals are digitized to enable lung volumes to be calculated. The machine operator can then open or close the valves to specify the duration of active breath-hold. This enables the lung tumour to only be irradiated when in the desired position to ensure tumour coverage at all times.

A further method to measure and account for lung and tumour motion in radiotherapy is 4D-CT data acquisition and planning. A 3D CT volume of the tumour and lung are taken while the patient breathes freely, with the couch in the same position. The CT images are then assigned a position in the respiratory cycle based on position of skin surface markers. When the newly positioned images are played on a continuous loop the result is a movie of the tumour and lung through their excursion on a respiratory cycle. Using modelling technology based on non-rigid registration algorithms the quality of this moving image can be improved. This is an area of current research and sophisticated 4D CT acquisition techniques will be used in radiotherapy planning and treatment delivery in the future [40–42]. Any system that is ultimately used successfully must be reproducible and accurate, be acceptable for wide patient acceptance and comfort and be practical to use in a busy clinical setting.

Conclusion

Radiotherapy is an integral part of the management of lung cancer patients. It is used in the radical and palliative setting, in conjunction with chemotherapy or surgery or as a single modality treatment. It is generally well tolerated by patients, although treatment courses can be long. Exciting research dedicated to improving radiotherapy planning and delivery is currently taking place worldwide to further develop radiation techniques. This in turn will lead to optimization of lung cancer management in the future.

REFERENCES

1. Brennan, P., Bray, I. (2002). Recent trends and future directions for lung cancer mortality in Europe. *BJC*, **87**, 43–8.
2. Gregor, A., Cull, A., Stephens, R. J., *et al.* (1997). Prophylactic cranial irradiation is indicated following complete response to induction therapy in small cell lung cancer: results of a multicentre randomised trial. United Kingdom Coordinating Committee for Cancer Research (UKCCCR) and the European Organization for Research and Treatment of Cancer (EORTC). *Eur J Cancer*, **33**, 1752–8.
3. Auperin, A., Arriagada, R., Pignon, J. P., *et al.* (1999). Prophylactic cranial irradiation for patients with small-cell lung cancer in complete remission. Prophylactic Cranial Irradiation Overview Collaborative Group. *N Engl J Med*, **341**, 476–844.
4. Devereux, S., *et al.* (1997). Immediate side effects of large fraction radiotherapy. *Clin Oncol*, **9**, 96–9.

5. Rees, G. J., Devrell, C. E., Barley, V. L., et al. (1997). Palliative radiotherapy for lung cancer: two versus five fractions. *Clin Oncol (R Coll Radiol)*, **9**(2), 90−5.

6. Dillman, R. O., Hendon, J., Seagren, S. L., et al. (1996). Improved survival in stage III non-small-cell lung cancer: seven-year follow-up of cancer and leukemia group B (CALGB) 8433 trial. *J Natl Cancer Inst*, **88**(17), 1210−5.

7. Sause, W. T., et al. (1995). Radiation Therapy Oncology Group 88−08 and Eastern Cooperative Oncology Group (ECOG) 4588: preliminary results of a phase III trial in regionally advanced unresectable non-small cell lung cancer. *J Natl Cancer Inst*, **87**, 198−205.

8. Furuse, K., Fukuoka, M., Kawahara, M., et al. (1999). Phase III study of concurrent versus sequential thoracic radiotherapy in combination with mitomycin, vindesine, and cisplatin in unresectable stage III non-small-cell lung cancer. *J Clin Oncol*, **17**(9), 2692−9.

9. Belani, C. P., Choy, H., Bonomi, P., et al. (2005). Combined chemoradiotherapy regimens of paclitaxel and carboplatin for locally advanced non-small-cell lung cancer: a randomized phase II locally advanced multi-modality protocol. *J Clin Oncol*, **23**(25), 5883−91. Epub 2005 Aug 8. Erratum in: *J Clin Oncol.* 2006 Apr 20; **24**(12): 1966.

10. Komaki, R., Seiferheld, W., Ettinger, D., et al. (2002). Randomised Phase II chemotherapy and radiotherapy trial for patients with locally advanced inoperable non-small cell lung cancer: long-term follow-up of RTOG 92−04. *Int J Radiation Oncology Biol Phys*, **53**(3), 548−57.

11. PORT Meta-analysis Trialists Group (1998). Post-operative radiotherapy in non-small cell lung cancer: a systematic review of individual patient data from nine randomised trials. *Lancet*, **352**, 257−63.

12. PORT Meta-analysis Trialists Group. (2003). Postoperative radiotherapy for non-small cell lung cancer. *Cochrane Database Syst Rev*, (1), CD002142. Review.

13. Zhang, H. X., Yin, W. B., Zhang, L. J., et al. (1989). Curative radiotherapy of early operable non-small cell lung cancer. *Radiotherapy Oncol*, **14**, 89−94.

14. Sibley, G. S., Jamieson, T. A., Marks, L. B., et al. (1998). Radiotherapy alone for medically inoperable Stage I non-small cell lung cancer: The Duke experience. *Int J Radiation Oncology Biol Phys*, **40**, 149−54.

15. Singh, A., Lockett, M., Bradley, J., et al. (2003). Predictors radiation-induced esophageal toxicity in patients with non-small cell lung cancer treated with three-dimensional conformal radiotherapy. *Int J Radiation Oncology Biol Phys*, **55**, 337−41.

16. Bradley, J., Thorstad, W. L., Mutic, S., et al. (2004). Impact of FDG-PET on radiation therapy volume delineation in non-small-cell lung cancer. *Int J Radiation Oncology Biol Phys*, **59**(1), 78−86.

17. Withers, H. R., Taylor, J. M. G., Maciejewski, B. (1998). The hazard of accelerated tumour clonogen repopulation during radiotherapy. *Acta Oncol*, **27**, 131−46.

18. Baumann, M., Liertz, C., Barisch, H., et al. (1994). Impact of overall treatment time of fractionated irradiation on local control of human FaDu squamous cell carcinoma in nude mice. *Radiother Oncol*, **32**, 137−43.

19. Saunders, M. I., Dische, S., Barrett, A., *et al.* (1996). Randomised multicentre trials of Continuous hyperfractionated accelerated radiotherapy (CHART) versus conventional radiotherapy in head and neck cancer and non-small cell lung cancer: an interim report. *Brit J Cancer*, **73**, 1455–62.

20. Saunders, M. I., Dische, S., Barrett, A., *et al.* (1999). Continuous hyperfractionated accelerated radiotherapy (CHART) versus conventional radiotherapy in non-small cell lung cancer: mature data from the randomised multicentre trial. *Radiother Oncol*, **52**, 137–47.

21. Gebitekin, C., Gupta, N. K., Satur, C. M., *et al.* (1994). Fate of patients with residual tumour at the bronchial resection margin. *Eur J Cardiothorac Surg*, **8**(7), 339–42; discussion 342–4.

22. Massard, G., Doddoli, C., Gasser, B., *et al.* (2000). Prognostic implications of a positive bronchial resection margin. *Eur J Cardiothorac Surg*, **17**(5), 557–65.

23. Pignon, J. P., Arriagada, R., Ihde, D. C., *et al.* (1992). A meta-analysis of thoracic radiotherapy for small-cell lung cancer. *N Engl J Med*, **327**, 1618–24.

24. Warde, P., Payne, D. (1992). Does thoracic irradiation improve survival and local control in limited-stage small-cell carcinoma of the lung? *A meta-analysis J Clin Oncol*, **10**, 890–95.

25. Coy, P., Hodson, I., Payne, D. G., *et al.* (1988). The effect of dose of thoracic irradiation on recurrence in patients with limited stage small cell lung cancer. Initial results of a Canadian Multicenter Randomized Trial. *Int J Radiat Oncol Biol Phys*, **14**(2), 219–26.

26. Gregor, A., Drings, P., Burghouts, J., *et al.* (1997). Randomized trial of alternating versus sequential radiotherapy/chemotherapy in limited-disease patients with small-cell lung cancer: a European Organization for Research and Treatment of Cancer Lung Cancer Cooperative Group Study. *J Clin Oncol*, **15**(8), 2840–9.

27. Turrisi, A., Kim, K., Blum, R., *et al.* (1999). Twice-daily compared with once-daily thoracic radiotherapy in limited small-cell lung cancer treated concurrently with cisplatin and etoposide. *N Engl J Med*, **340**(4), 265–71.

28. Fried, D. B., Morris, D. E., Poole, C., *et al.* Systematic review evaluating the timing of thoracic radiation therapy in combined modality therapy for limited stage small cell lung cancer. *J Clin Oncol*, **22**(23), 4837–45.

29. Healey, E. A., Abner, A. (1995). Thoracic and cranial radiotherapy for limited-stage small cell lung cancer. *Chest*, **107**(6 Suppl), 2595–2545.

30. Jeremic, B., Shibamato, Y., Nikolic, N., *et al.* (1999). Role of radiation therapy in the combined-modality treatment of patients with extensive disease small-cell lung cancer: A randomized study. *J Clin Oncol*, **17**(7), 2092–9.

31. Landberg, T., Charaudra, J., Dobbs, H. J., *et al.* (1993). *Prescribing, recording and reporting photon beam therapy.* Bethesda, Maryland: ICRU. International Commission on Radiation Units and Measurements ICRU Report 50.

32. Landberg, T., Charaudra, J., Dobbs, H. J., *et al.* (1999). International Commission on Radiation Units and Measurements ICRU Report 62, Supplement to ICRU Report 50.

33. Grills, I. S., Yan, D., Martinez, A. A., *et al.* (2003). Potential for reduced toxicity and dose escalation in the treatment of inoperable non-small cell lung cancer: a comparison of intensity-modulated radiation therapy (IMRT), 3D conformal radiation and elective nodal irradiation. *Int J Radiat Oncol Biol Phys*, **57**(3), 875—90.

34. Murshed, H., Lin, H., Zhongxing, L., *et al.* (2004) Dose and volume reduction for normal lung using intensity-modulated radiotherapy for advanced-stage non-small cell lung cancer. *Int J Radiation Oncology Biol Phys*, **58**, 1258—67.

35. Armstrong, J. G. (1998). Target volume definition for three-dimensional conformal radiation therapy of lung cancer. *British Journal of Radiology*, 587—94.

36. Senan, S., van Sornsen de Koste, J., Samon, M., *et al.* (1999). Evaluation of a target contouring protocol for 3D conformal radiotherapy in non-small cell lung cancer. *Radiother Oncol*, **53**, 247—55.

37. Kudo, H. D., Hill, B. C. (1996). Respiration gated radiotherapy treatment: A technical study. *Phys Med Biol*, **41**, 83—91.

38. Vedam, S. S., Keall, P. J., Kini, V. R., *et al.* (2001). Determining parameters for respiration-gated radiotherapy. *Med Phys*, **28**, 2139—46.

39. Wong, J. W., Sharpe, M. B., Jaffray, D. A., *et al.* (1999). The use of active breathing control (ABC) to reduce margin for breathing motion. *Int J Radiation Oncology Biol Phys*, **44**(4), 911—9.

40. Cheung, P. C., Sixel, K. E., Tirona, R., *et al.* (2003). Reproducibility of lung tumour position and reduction of lung mass within the planning target volume using active breathing control (ABC). *Int J Radiation Oncology Biol Phys*, **57**(5), 1437—42.

41. Low, D. A., Nystrom, M., Kalinin, E., *et al.* (2003). A method for the reconstruction of four dimensional synchronised CT scans acquired during free breathing. *Med Phys*, **30**(6), 1254—63.

42. Vedam, S. S., Keall, P. J., Kini, V. R., *et al.* (2003). Acquiring a four dimensional computed tomography dataset using an external respiratory signal. *Phys Med Biol*, **48**, 45—62.

43. Keall, P. J., Joshi, S., Vedam, S. S., *et al.* (2005) Four-dimensional radiotherapy planning for DMLC-based respiratory motion tracking. *Med Phys*, **32**(4), 942—51.

44. Medical Research Council Lung Cancer Working Party. (1991). Inoperable non-small cell lung cancer: A Medical Research Council randomised trial of palliative radiotherapy of two fractions or ten fractions. *Br J Cancer*, **63**, 265—70.

45. Medical Research Council Lung Cancer Working Party (1992). A Medical Research Council randomised trial of palliative radiotherapy of two fractions or a single fraction in patients with inoperable non-small cell lung cancer (NSCLC) and poor performance status. *Br J Cancer*, **65**, 934—41.

46. Macbeth, F. R., *et al.* (1996). Randomised trial of palliative two-fraction versus more intensive 13-fractionradiotherapy for patients with inoperable non-small cell lung cancer and good performance status. Medical Research Council Lung Cancer Working Party. *Clin Oncol*, **8**, 167—75.

47. Erridge, S. C., Gaze, M. N., Price, A., *et al.* (2005). Symptom control and Quality of Life in people with lung cancer: a randomised trial of two palliative radiotherapy fractionation schedules. *Clin Oncol*, **17**(1), 61−7.

48. Toy, E., Macbeth, F. R., Cohen, B., *et al.* (2003). Palliative thoracic radiotherapy for non-small cell lung cancer: a systematic review. *Am J Clin Oncol*, **26**(2), 112−20.

49. Ekberg, L., Holmberg, O., Wittgren, *et al.* (1998). What margins should be added to the clinical target volume in radiotherapy treatment planning for lung cancer. *Radiother Oncol*, **48**(1), 71−7.

50. Stevens, C., Munden, R., Forster, K., *et al.* (2001). Respiratory-driven lung tumour motion is independent of tumour size, tumour location and pulmonary function. *Int J Radiation Oncology Biol Phys*, **51**, 62−8.

51. Steel, G. (1997). *Basic Clinical radiobiology* (2nd Edition).

52. De Vita, V., Hellman, S., Rosenberg, S. (2001). *Cancer Principles & Practice of Oncology* (6th Edition).

9

Surgery for Lung Cancer

Andrew Chukwuemeka and Michael T. Marrinan

Department of Cardiothoracic Surgery, King's College Hospital, London, UK

Introduction

Surgical resection has, for most of the past century, been considered the main hope for cure in patients with non-small cell lung cancer (NSCLC). However, it is fair to state that this view is changing. Although surgery may be curative, it is salutary to note that operative treatment is a viable option in only around 10% of patients. The reasons for this are relatively straightforward: most patients have advanced stage disease at presentation, and impaired pulmonary function or co-morbidity preclude major surgery [1]. Moreover, the success rate for resection in this select group is generally low and it must be noted that even in stage I disease, 5-year survival is only 65% after surgery [2, 3].

The limited scope and success of potentially curative surgical resection may be compared historically with the even more modest successes of radiotherapy and chemotherapy. However, there has been something of a recent revolution; significant improvements in outcomes (with chemotherapy in particular), have offered new hope to patients with lung cancer and have helped to clarify and refine the role of surgical resection for primary lung cancer. Indeed, far from reducing the role of surgery, this welcome and long overdue improvement in survival with combined treatment modalities is likely to increase the role of surgery by expanding the accepted clinico-pathological stages likely to benefit from resection.

Radiologist and Surgeon Working Together

An obvious but important tenet of lung cancer surgery is that resection is only effective for localized disease. Plainly, surgery is of limited value when disease is advanced. Indeed, there is a valid view that surgery undertaken in the presence of disseminated disease may hasten death. If the role of surgery is to excize localized disease then the key role of the radiologist is to identify whether the disease is in fact localized.

The radiologist is intrinsic to the primary diagnosis and pre-operative staging of lung cancer. Furthermore, where appropriate, the radiologist may undertake image-guided percutaneous needle biopsy of suspicious lesions. The increase in incidence of peripheral adenocarcinoma of the lung [4] has driven the need for percutaneous needle biopsy for diagnosis, as many of these lesions are not amenable to bronchoscopic diagnosis.

Because cigarette smoking is the principal aetiological agent in the causation of lung cancer it comes as no surprize that many patients have co-morbidity due to cardiorespiratory disease (Fig. 9.1). The radiologist has an important role in identifying and characterizing co-morbidity particularly pulmonary disease. Fibrosing lung diseases in particular are associated with a significantly increased risk when resection is undertaken for primary lung cancer. Unfortunately, lung cancer is more common in this group and a full radiological assessment of patients with pulmonary fibrosis is essential before the decision to operate is made.

Staging and the Decision to Operate

In deciding whether to offer surgery to a patient with NSCLC an assessment of 'resectability' (should the tumour be removed?) and 'operability' (will the patient survive the resection?) must be made. Current evidence suggests that surgical resection, with curative intent, is appropriate only for stages I and II NSCLC in which it is believed that the attendant operative morbidity and mortality are acceptable [2, 3]. Resection should be anatomical wherever possible, which usually means lobectomy or bi-lobectomy and less frequently pneumonectomy. The survival benefit of lesser procedures such as wedge resection or segmentectomy is reduced significantly when compared with anatomical resection [5]. Nevertheless, a significant number of patients with advanced co-morbidity or severely impaired pulmonary function, who would not withstand a lobectomy, may still be suitable for wedge resection and may derive some benefit from this less extensive procedure.

Emerging Trends in Surgical Treatment

A trend is emerging for surgery in the treatment of lung cancer. It is very likely that it will increasingly be combined with neo-adjuvant and adjuvant chemotherapy

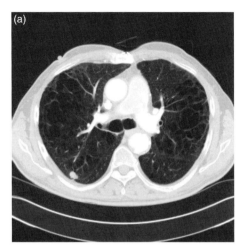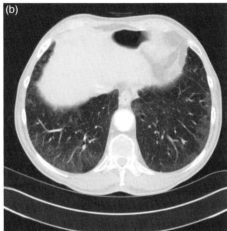

Figure 9.1 Two images from a patient with a peripheral squamous cell carcinoma of the lung cancer. (a) CT at the level of the carina demonstrates a small spiculated lesion in the posterior segment of the right upper lobe. There is extensive centrilobular emphysema. (b) Image through the lower zones demonstrates a fine subpleural reticular pattern and ground-glass opacification indicating established interstitial fibrosis

and occasionally radiotherapy. It is hoped that the acceptable stages for surgical resection will thereby be increased. The role of neo-adjuvant chemotherapy in early stage lung cancer will be defined in the next few years and should lead to improved outcomes.

Down-staging of Disease

For patients with stage III NSCLC there remains controversy about the most appropriate management. There are a lack of meaningful large-scale randomized trials and stage III NSCLC also comprises a relatively heterogeneous group. For instance, Stage IIIA includes patients with metastases to ipsilateral mediastinal nodes (N2) as well as those with T3N1 disease, whilst stage IIIB comprises patients with any T4, any N, M0 tumours and those with N3M0 tumours. The majority of patients with stage IIIA disease will, however, have N2 disease and it is in this particular subset that the possibility of 'downstaging' N2 nodes by neo-adjuvant chemotherapy and radiotherapy may prove beneficial and allow for subsequent successful resection of residual disease with a potential for cure.

Stage T1-3 N2M0 Non-small Cell Lung Cancer

A number of phase II non-randomized clinical trials have attempted to establish the utility of neo-adjuvant chemotherapy and radiotherapy in this subset of patients. Martini and colleagues, for example, showed significantly improved survival with induction chemotherapy for patients who had bulky mediastinal disease [6]. A number of small randomized trials also support the use of neo-adjuvant chemotherapy in this group of patients. In one study, patients were randomized to either surgery alone or three cycles of induction chemotherapy and showed a significant improvement in two year and five year survival [7]. Simialrly, Roth and co-workers were able to demonstrate a survival benefit for induction chemotherapy in their patient cohort [8]. Despite these promising data, it must be remembered that all the above trials were conducted on relatively small cohorts generally with chemotherapy regimes that are now considered outdated. However, these earlier studies emphasize the need for larger studies that are currently in progress (EORTC 08941 and NAI 0139). It should also be noted that neo-adjuvant chemotherapy has potential disadvantages delaying control of the primary tumour and significantly increase surgical morbidity and mortality [9]. This increase in operative morbidity and mortality may be compounded when pre-operative radiotherapy has also been given. Thus, current practice is that neo-adjuvant chemotherapy or chemo-radiotherapy for stage III NSCLC should only be used in the context of a clinical trial whenever possible.

Stage IIIB Non-small Cell Lung Cancer

Surgery is only indicated for carefully selected patients with T4 N0-1 M0 tumours and the role of neo-adjuvant therapy or chemo-radiotherapy is still being evaluated. Patients with stage T4N1M0 disease, due solely to the presence of a satellite tumour nodule, may benefit from surgery with a five-year survival of 20% [10]. In tumours staged as T4N0M0 due to carinal involvement, a 20% 5-year survival can be achieved with resection although such surgery is associated with an operative mortality of 10−15% [11]. Superior sulcus (Pancoast) tumours that are not extensively locally invasive are amenable to surgical resection in the absence of mediastinal lymph node involvement; the use of induction chemo-radiotherapy has been shown to improve survival [12].

Broncho-Alveolar Cell Carcinoma

Special mention is made of this tumour which occurs in two main forms. Bronchoalveolar commonly presents as a diffuse tumour and, accordingly, surgery is seldom indicated due to the propensity for multifocal metastatic spread within the lungs [13]. Broncho-alveolar cell carcinoma can also occur, less frequently, as a nodular tumour, in which case surgery may be recommended based on the same stage criteria as for the other NSCLCs.

Small Cell Lung Cancer

Surgical resection, as an option in the treatment of small cell lung cancer (SCLC), was abandoned in the 1970s as it was abundantly clear that long-term survival for these patients was dismal: fewer than 5% of patients were alive at five years [14]. More recently, the introduction of multi-modality treatment which includes surgery for stage I SCLC has achieved five year survival rates of 35–40% and surgery can now be recommended for the very small number of patients who have peripheral small cell tumours with no nodal involvement [15]. Due to the rapid doubling time of small cell lung cancer, surgery should be undertaken with dispatch.

Positron Emission Tomography

The sensitivity and specificity of positron emission tomography (PET) scanning in lung cancer and the general utility of this investigation are dealt with in a separate chapter in this volume. However, it is pertinent to highlight four specific aspects of the use of PET in lung cancer which are of particular interest to surgeons. First, it should be emphasized that SUVs as low as 1.5 may not exclude cancer and are in fact a common finding in adenocarcinoma of the lung. Second, the potential for finding unexpected metastases is a real benefit of using PET scanning as a pre-operative diagnostic tool, thus avoiding unwarranted surgery. It is the practice in our unit to obtain whole-body PET in all elective patients being considered for surgical resection. Third, particular care must be taken of negative results of PET scanning where the patient may have a neuro-endocrine tumour. In this situation, octreotide scanning may be a more sensitive procedure. Finally, there is a growing body of evidence to suggest that the prognosis is poor in patients who have an exceptionally high SUV even though their staging suggests that they would be suitable for surgical resection [16]. In the absence of robust evidence for this, our group has taken the view that a course of neo adjuvant chemotherapy is appropriate. It is likely that this aspect of surgical selection will be clarified in the next few years.

Conclusion

Surgical resection of localized non-disseminated NSCLC remains the standard of care but is limited in applicability. Combined treatment with chemotherapy or chemo-radiation and surgical resection may prove to be beneficial for patients presenting with more advanced stage NSCLC.

REFERENCES

1. Royal College of Physicians Joint Specialty Committee for Medical Oncology. The cancer patient's physician: recommendations for the development of medical oncology in England and Wales. London: Royal College of Physicians, 2000.
2. Naruke, T., Goya, T., Tsuchiya, R., *et al.* (1988). Prognosis and survival in resected lung carcinoma based on the new international staging system. *Thorac Cardiocasc Surg*, **96**, 440–7.
3. Mountain, C. F. (1997). Revisions in the international system for staging lung cancer. *Chest*, **111**, 1710–7.
4. Rusch, V. W., Ginsberg, R. J. (1999). Lung tumours. In Schwartz S I (ed): *Principles of Surgery*, 7th ed. New York, McGraw-Hill.
5. Ginsberg, R. J., Rubenstein, L. V. (1996). A randomised comparative trial of lobectomy vs. limited resection for patients with T1N0 non-small cell lung cancer. *Lung Cancer*, **7**, 83–8.
6. Martini, N., Kris, M. G., Flehinger, B. J., *et al.* (1993). Preoperative chemotherapy for stage IIIA (N2) lung cancer: The Sloan-Kettering experience in 136 patients. *Ann Thorac Surg*, **55**, 992–8.
7. Rosell, R., Gomez-Codina, J., Camps, C., *et al.* (1999). Preresectional chemotherapy in stage IIIA non-small cell lung cancer. *Lung Cancer*, **26**, 7–14.
8. Roth, J. A., Atkinson, E. N., Fosella, F., *et al.* (1998). Long-term follow-up of patients enrolled in a randomised trial comparing perioperative chemotherapy and surgery. *Lung Cancer*, **21**, 1–6.
9. Robert, J. R., Eustis, C., DeVore, R. F., *et al.* (2001). Induction chemotherapy increases perioperative complications in patients undergoing resection for non-small cell lung cancer. *Ann Thorac Surg*, **72**, 885–8.

10. Deslauriers, J., Brisson, J., Cartier, R., *et al.* (1989). Carcinoma of the lung: evaluation of satellite nodules as a factor influencing prognosis after resection. *Thorac Cardiovasc Surg*, **97**, 504–12.

11. Jett, J. R., Scott, W. J., Rivera, M. P., Sause, W. T. (2003). Guidelines on treatment of stage IIIB non-small cell lung cancer. *Chest*, **123**, 221–5S.

12. Rusch, V. W., Giroux, D. J., Kraut, M. J., *et al.* (2001). Induction chemoradiation and surgical resection for non-small cell lung carcinomas of the superior sulcus: initial results of Southwest Oncology Group Trial 9416 (Intergroup Trial 0160) *J Thorac Cardiovasc Surg*, **121**(3), 472–83.

13. Laskin, J. J., Sandler, A. B., Johnson, D. H. (2005). Redefining bronchioloalveolar carcinoma. *Semin Oncol*, **32**(3), 329–35.

14. Fox, W., Scadding, J. G. (1973). Medical Research Council comparative trial of surgery and radiotherapy for primary treatment of small-celled or oat-celled carcinoma of bronchus: tenyear follow-up. *Lancet*, **2**, 63–5.

15. Rea, F., Callegaro, D., Favaretto, A., *et al.* (1998). Long term results of surgery and chemotherapy in small cell lung cancer. *Eur J Cardiothorac Surg*, **14**, 398–402.

16. Dhital, K., Saunders, C. A., Seed, P. T., O'Doherty, M. J., Dussek, J. (2000). (18)F Fluoro-deoxyglucose positron emission tomography and its prognostic value in lung cancer. *Eur J Cardiothorac Surg*, **18**, 425–8.

Index